INTERMITTENT FASTING Series

The Comprehensive Guide to Eat Healthy and Feel Better Following this Lifestyle with complete diet plan.

By Melissa White

3

BOOK1

BOOK2

INTERMITTENT FASTING DIET PLAN

intermittent fasting is the best
way to loss weight step-by-step

Chapter 1. Mechanism of Action of Intermittent Fasting Diet Plan

Intermittent fasting is a form of eating plan in which you alternate between fasting and eating on a regular basis. Intermittent fasting has been shown in studies to help people lose weight and avoid or even cure disease.

Many diets emphasize when to eat, but intermittent fasting emphasizes what to eat. When you fast intermittently, you only feed at certain times of the day. Fasting for a set number of hours per day or consuming just one meal a couple of times a week will aid fat loss. Scientific evidence also suggests that there are certain health benefits. Now we discuss the mechanism of action of intermittent fasting:

1.1 The Fed State of Intermittent Fasting

After a meal, the body is in the absorptive stage, or fed state, where it is digesting the food and absorbing the nutrients (catabolism exceeds anabolism). When you put food in your mouth, it is broken down into its constituent parts and consumed into the intestine, which is when digestion starts. Carbohydrate digestion starts in the mouth, while protein and fat digestion begins in the stomach and small intestine. The components of these carbohydrates, fats, and proteins pass the intestinal wall and reach the bloodstream (sugars and amino acids) or lymphatic system (fats). These systems move them from the intestines to the liver, adipose tissue, or muscle cells, where they are processed and stored.

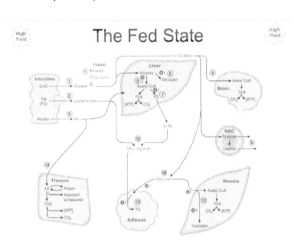

The Fed State

1.1.1 For How Long Fed State Lasts?

The absorptive or fed state will last up to 4 hours, depending on the amount and form of nutrients consumed. Food consumption and rising blood glucose levels cause pancreatic beta cells to release insulin into the bloodstream, where it begins the absorption of blood glucose by liver hepatocytes, as well as adipose and muscle cells. Glucose is converted to glucose-6-phosphate as soon as it enters these cells. This allows glucose to move from the bloodstream to the cells, where it is needed. Insulin also promotes glucose preservation as glycogen in the liver and muscle cells, where it can be used for the body's future energy needs. Insulin also encourages muscle protein synthesis. Muscle protein can be catabolized and used as food in times of hunger, as you'll see.

If you exert energy soon after eating, the dietary fats and sugars you just consumed will be stored and used for energy right away. If not, excess glucose is retained as glycogen in the liver and muscle cells, or as fat in the adipose tissue; excess dietary fat is often stored as triglycerides in the adipose tissue. The metabolic processes that occur in the body during the absorptive state.

1.1.2 The Processing of Fed State

In the fed or absorptive state following nutrients are processed:

Carbohydrates: are simple sugars that are transported to the liver and converted to glucose. The glucose is then transported to the bloodstream or transformed into glycogen and fat (triglyceride). Glycogen and fat would be retained as reserves for the post-absorptive condition in the liver and adipose tissue, respectively. The excess glucose is either absorbed by body cells or retained as glycogen in skeletal muscle.

Triglycerides: Chylomicrons, the primary product of fat digestion, are first hydrolyzed and broken down into fatty acids and glycerol by Lipoprotein lipase. They are able to freely move through capillary walls as a result of this. The majority of it will be converted to triglycerides and deposited in adipose tissue. Adipose cells, skeletal muscles, and hepatocytes use the remainder for energy. Other body cells will start to use triglycerides as energy sources in a low carb setting.

Amino Acids: The liver converts amino acids to keto acids, which are then used in the Krebs cycle to generate ATP. It's also possible that they'll be converted to fat stores. Some are used to produce plasma proteins, but the majority pass

16

through the liver sinusoids and are used to construct proteins by body cells.

After eating a meal or snack, you enter the fed state. Your body begins to break down and consume the nutrients from the food as soon as you eat it. This digested material's components reach your bloodstream, causing blood glucose levels to increase. The increase in glucose causes your pancreas' beta cells to release insulin, which binds to receptors in your cells, causing them to open and let glucose in.

1.1.3 Role of Glucose

Three things happen once glucose enters the cells:

1. The cells use it as a direct source of energy.

2. Converted to glycogen and processed for later use in your liver and muscles.

3. Converted to triglycerides, which are then processed as fat in your body.

Until all of the digested content has passed through the gastrointestinal tract, you are legally fed. When you're in a federal state, you must:

• Insulin levels are high.

• Glucose levels are high.

• You are burning glucose for energy and storing fat.

A fed state usually lasts four hours after eating, depending on what you consume, but if you never go longer than four hours between meals or snacks, your body will still be in a fed state.

1.1.4 Breakdown to Simpler Units

Following a meal, various hydrolases in the brush border of the intestine break down carbohydrates to simple sugars, which are then imported into intestinal enterocytes through a sodium symporter. Amino acids (AAs) are broken down from proteins and imported into intestinal enterocytes through a sodium symport. The AAs and glucose are then absorbed into the bloodstream and transferred to the liver via the hepatic portal vein. The majority of lipids are packed into chylomicrons, which join lacteals and then enter the bloodstream through the thoracic duct.

Insulin is released from beta cells in the pancreatic islets when blood glucose and amino acid levels increase after a meal. Insulin is the main hormone that tells muscles, tissues, and cells what to do with the nutrients they've consumed during the absorptive state. Under the influence of growth hormone (GH) and androgens/estrogens, all tissues increase their intake and consumption of AAs and glucose, glucose for energy in part to fuel protein synthesis of the imported AAs.

Before the blood enters the inferior vena cava, the liver controls the levels of glucose and amino acids in the blood arriving at the hepatic portal vein, keeping glucose levels at or below 150 mg/dl after a meal. Hepatocytes transform glucose to glycogen (glycogenesis) until liver reserves are depleted (about 5% by weight), then use the glucose for energy (glycolysis).If there is still too much glucose in the blood, hepatocytes convert it to triglycerides, which are then exported in VLDLs and taken up by adipose tissues. Plasma amino acid levels (between 35 and 65 mg/dl) are also regulated by the liver, but not as specifically as glucose levels. Hepatocytes either use amino acids for protein synthesis or convert them to less available amino acids that are then circulated to other tissues for protein synthesis.

Insulin directs adipocytes to take up fatty acids and glycerol for triglyceride synthesis in adipose tissue (lipogenesis).

Amino acids are imported as required for protein synthesis, and glucose is taken up to fuel their synthesis.

1.2 The Post-absorptive State of Intermittent Fasting

When food has been digested, consumed, and processed, the post-absorptive condition, also known as fasting, occurs. Fasting overnight is normal, but missing meals during the day often puts the body in a post-absorptive condition. Initially, the body must depend on glycogen stored in the muscles. As glucose is consumed and used by the cells, blood glucose levels begin to fall. Insulin levels drop in response to a reduction in glucose. Collection of glycogen and triglycerides slows. Blood glucose levels must be held in the normal range of 80–120 mg/dL due to the demands of the tissues and organs. The hormone glucagon is released by the pancreas' alpha cells in response to a decrease in blood glucose levels. Glucagon works by inhibiting glycogen synthesis and stimulating the breakdown of stored glycogen back into glucose in liver cells. The liver releases this glucose for use by the peripheral tissues and the brain. Glucose levels in the blood begin to rise as a result. To replace the glucose that has been used by the peripheral tissues, gluconeogenesis will begin   in   the   liver.

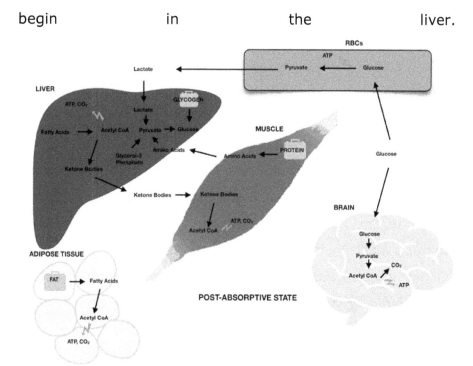

1.2.1 How Fats are processed?

Fats and proteins are processed as mentioned previously after ingestion of food; however, glucose processing differs slightly. Glucose is absorbed more readily in the peripheral tissues. After a long fast, the liver, which usually consumes and processes glucose, will not do so. After fasting, the gluconeogenesis that has been going on in the liver will begin to replenish the glycogen stocks that have been depleted. Excess glucose absorbed by the liver is transformed to triglycerides and fatty acids for long-term storage after these supplies have been replenished. The metabolic processes that occur in the body during the post-absorptive state.

The post-absorptive condition occurs when catabolism outnumbers anabolism in the body. The body must maintain homeostasis during the post-absorptive state, which it does through a variety of catabolic processes, including the breakdown of glycogen to glucose, triglycerides to gylcerol and fatty acids, proteins to amino acids, glycogen to pyruvate, and fatty acids to ketones. Since the central nervous system relies solely on glucose for energy, it's important that blood glucose levels remain stable. This is accomplished by secreting glucagon, which encourages the liver to degrade glucose storage. When plasma glucose concentrations fall too low, changes in neural activity begin to occur. Furthermore, the body begins to convert stored fatty acids into energy and ketone bodies.

1.2.2 Glycogen as a Source of Energy

After your food has been completely digested, consumed, and processed, you enter the fasted state, also known as the post-absorptive period. The digested materials have passed through the gastrointestinal tract, the glucose level in your bloodstream has stabilized, and your body is now relying on stored glycogen for energy. When blood glucose levels fall, insulin levels fall as well. The alpha cells in your pancreas release glucagon, a hormone that moves to the liver and aids in the conversion of glycogen back into glucose, to keep glucose levels between 70 and 99 milligrams per deciliter (the normal range for adults). The glucose then moves to your cells, giving your brain and tissues energy.

• When you're fasted, the insulin and glucose levels are both low.

• The body begins to use fat as a source of energy. You're losing weight.

Since the fed state lasts four hours and you normally don't enter the fasted state until four hours after your last meal, unless you time your food intake, your body is unlikely to enter this fat-burning state. This is one of the reasons why, even though they don't change anything else, many women lose weight and body fat when they begin intermittent fasting. Fasting puts the body into a fat-burning state that is difficult to achieve on a regular eating schedule.

1.2.3 What Cause the Increase of Fatty Acids?

Enterocytes avoid supplying glucose to the hepatic portal circulation as the absorptive state ends. Peripheral tissues continue to absorb glucose until plasma glucose levels fall below about 80 mg/dl, at which point hepatocytes begin to catabolize their glycogen stores (glycogenolysis) into glucose in response to the levels of glucagon (released by pancreatic islet alpha cells) and epinephrine, signaling the start of the post-absorptive state. After around four hours of liver glycogenolysis, liver reserves deplete and blood glucose levels drop (to about 70 mg/dl). The liver stabilizes glucose levels at this stage by undergoing gluconeogenesis, which is triggered by glucocorticoids released from the adrenal cortex. To power gluconeogenesis, the liver takes glycerol, lactate, and amino acids from the blood, as well as fatty acids. Increased circulating levels of glucocorticoids and epinephrine have caused circulating fatty acids and glycerol used for gluconeogenesis to be mobilized from adipose tissue. The liver becomes increasingly involved in the import of amino acids for gluconeogenesis (from glucogenic AAs) and ketogenesis (ketogenesis) as the time of the post-absorptive state increases (from ketogenic AAs).

Peripheral tissues decrease their dependence on circulating glucose and increase their reliance on lipids and ketones as circulating levels of these compounds rise during the post-absorptive state. Neural tissues rely on glucose until glucose levels are inadequate to satisfy their energetic demands, at which point they must rely on circulating ketones.

1.3 Starvation Mode in Intermittent Fasting

At the point when the body is denied of sustenance for an all-inclusive timeframe, it goes into "endurance mode." The main goal for endurance is to give sufficient glucose or fuel to the mind. The subsequent need is the protection of amino acids for proteins. Accordingly, the body utilizes ketones to fulfill the energy needs of the cerebrum and other glucose-subordinate organs, and to keep up proteins in the cells. Since glucose levels are low during starvation, glycolysis will close off in cells that can utilize elective powers. Muscles, for example, can switch from glucose to unsaturated fats as a source of energy. As recently clarified, unsaturated fats can be changed over into acetyl CoA and handled through the Krebs cycle to make ATP. Pyruvate, lactate, and alanine from muscle cells are not changed over into acetyl CoA and utilized in the Krebs cycle, however are traded to the liver to be utilized in the combination of glucose. Glycerol from unsaturated fats can be liberated and used as a hotspot for gluconeogenesis as malnutrition progresses and more glucose is needed.

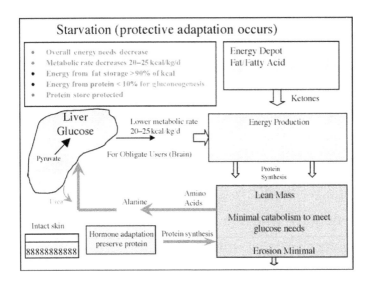

1.3.1 What will happen after few days of Starvation?

Following a few days of starvation, ketone bodies become the significant wellspring of fuel for the heart and different organs. As starvation proceeds, unsaturated fats and fatty substance stores are utilized to make ketones for the body. This forestalls the proceeded with breakdown of proteins that fill in as carbon hotspots for gluconeogenesis. When these stores are completely drained, proteins from muscles are delivered and separated for glucose amalgamation. In general endurance is subject to the measure of fat and protein put away in the body.

In case you're new to skipping suppers, your first idea might be "However what might be said about starvation mode?" Numerous individuals say that you will enter starvation mode in the event that you avoid a supper or don't eat frequently enough. That is the place where eating a few little suppers, rather than three enormous ones, came from. Truth be told, when somebody who's consuming less calories arrives at a weight reduction level, intermittently the exhortation is that they're not eating enough and just need to eat all the more regularly to keep the body from entering starvation mode. In any case, it doesn't work very like that. Starvation mode, the specialized name for versatile thermogenesis, is your body's physiological reaction to an extreme calorie shortfall, not avoiding a couple of dinners to a great extent. At the point when you seriously confine calories, your body deciphers that as a danger to endurance. Thus, your focal sensory system and your chemicals cooperate to hinder your digestion and save energy so that it's harder to lose muscle to fat ratio. In the event that you stay in this calorie-limited state for a really long time, it can cause hormonal awkward nature and expanded trouble keeping a sound weight. Now, it currently gets delegated metabolic harm a physiological condition that can cause considerably more extreme hormonal awkward nature (particularly with the appetite chemicals) and muscle misfortune. Since intermittent fasting is definitely not an extreme limitation of calories, it doesn't trigger versatile thermogenesis. It really does the inverse. At the point when you center on feast timing, as opposed to serious calorie limitation, it helps balance chemicals, save slender bulk, and improve your digestion. At the point when done right, intermittent fasting can even opposite metabolic harm and metabolic condition.

Starvation is an extreme insufficiency in caloric energy consumption, beneath the level expected to keep a creature's life. It is the most limit type of unhealthiness. In people, drawn out starvation can cause lasting organ harm and in the long run, passing. The term inanition alludes to the manifestations and impacts of starvation. Starvation may likewise be utilized as a methods for torment or execution.

1.3.2 Excessive Starvation may be a Danger to Health

As indicated by the World Health Organization, hunger is the single gravest danger to the world's general wellbeing. The WHO likewise expresses that unhealthiness is by a wide margin the greatest supporter of kid mortality, present in portion, all things considered. Under nutrition is a contributory factor in the passing of 3.1 million youngsters under five consistently. Figures on real starvation are hard to get, however as indicated by the Food and Agriculture Organization, the less serious state of undernourishment right now influences around 842 million individuals, or around one out of eight (12.5%) individuals in the total populace.

The swelled stomach addresses a type of lack of healthy sustenance called kwashiorkor. The specific pathogenesis of kwashiorkor isn't clear, as at first it was thought to identify with abstains from food high in sugars (for example maize) however low in protein. While numerous patients have low egg whites, this is believed to be an outcome of the condition. Potential causes, for example, aflatoxin harming, oxidative pressure, resistant deregulation, and modified gut micro biota have been proposed. Treatment can help relieve manifestations like the imagined weight reduction and muscle squandering, anyway anticipation is of most extreme significance.

The early phases of starvation sway mental status and practices. These manifestations appear as bad tempered state of mind, weakness, inconvenience concentrating, and distraction with food contemplations. Individuals with those manifestations will in general be quickly drawn off-track and have no energy.

As starvation advances, the actual indications set in. The circumstance of these indications relies upon age, size, and in general wellbeing. It generally requires days to weeks, and incorporates shortcoming, quick pulse, shallow breaths that are eased back, thirst, and clogging. There may likewise be looseness of the bowels sometimes. The eyes start to soak in and glass over. The muscles start to decrease and muscle squandering sets in. One noticeable sign in kids is a swollen tummy. Skin extricates and turns pale in shading, and there might be expanding of the feet and lower legs.

1.3.3 Side effects of Starvation

Side effects of starvation may likewise show up as a debilitated insusceptible framework, moderate injury mending, and helpless reaction to disease. Rashes may create on the skin. The body coordinates any supplements accessible to keeping organs working.

Different impacts of starvation may include: gallstones, sporadic or missing periods in ladies.

The manifestations of starvation appear in three phases. Stage one and two can appear in anybody that skips suppers, abstains from food, and goes through fasting. Stage three is more serious, can be lethal, and results from long haul starvation.

Stage one: When suppers are skipped, the body starts to keep up glucose levels by delivering glycogen in the liver and separating put away fat and protein. The liver can give glycogen to the initial not many hours. From that point onward, the body starts to separate fat and protein. Unsaturated fats are utilized by the body as a fuel hotspot for muscles, however bring down the measure of glucose that gets to the mind. Another substance that comes from unsaturated fats is glycerol. It tends to be utilized like glucose for energy, however ultimately runs out.

Stage two: Phase two can keep going for up to weeks all at once. In this stage, the body for the most part utilizes put away fat for energy. The breakdown happens in the liver and transforms fat into ketones. In the wake of fasting has continued for multi week, the mind will utilize these ketones and any extra glucose. Utilizing ketones brings down the requirement for glucose, and the body eases back the breakdown of proteins.

Stage three: By this point, the fat stores are gone and the body starts to go to put away protein for energy. This implies it needs to separate muscle tissues which are loaded with protein; the muscles separate rapidly. Protein is fundamental for our cells to work appropriately, and when it runs out, the cells can at this point don't work.

The reason for death because of starvation is normally a disease, or the aftereffect of tissue breakdown. The body can't acquire sufficient energy to fend off microscopic organisms and infections. The signs toward the end stages include: hair shading misfortune, skin chipping, growing in the furthest points, and a swelled tummy. Despite the fact that they may feel hunger, individuals in the end-phase of starvation are generally unfit to eat sufficient food.

With a commonplace high-starch diet, the human body depends on free blood glucose as its essential fuel source. Glucose can be gotten straightforwardly from dietary sugars and by the breakdown of different starches. Without dietary sugars and carbs, glucose is acquired from the breakdown of put away glycogen. Glycogen is a promptly available capacity type of glucose, put away in outstanding amounts in the liver and skeletal muscle.

After the fatigue of the glycogen save, and for the following 2–3 days, unsaturated fats become the foremost metabolic fuel. From the start, the mind keeps on utilizing glucose. On the off chance that a non-cerebrum tissue is utilizing unsaturated fats as its metabolic fuel, the utilization of glucose in a similar tissue is turned off. Subsequently, when unsaturated fats are being separated for energy, the entirety of the leftover glucose is made accessible for use by the cerebrum.

Following 2 or 3 days of fasting, the liver starts to blend ketone bodies from forerunners acquired from unsaturated fat breakdown. The cerebrum utilizes these ketone bodies as fuel, subsequently cutting its necessity for glucose. In the wake of fasting for 3 days, the mind gets 30% of its energy from ketone bodies. Following 4 days, this may increment to 70% or more. Subsequently, the creation of ketone bodies cuts the cerebrum's glucose necessity from 80 g each day to 30 g each day, about 35% of ordinary, with 65% got from ketone bodies. In any case, of the cerebrum's excess 30 g prerequisite, 20 g each day can be delivered by the liver from glycerol (itself a result of fat breakdown). This actually leaves a shortage of around 10 g of glucose each day that should be provided from another source; this other source will be the body's own proteins.

After depletion of fat stores, the cells in the body start to separate protein. This deliveries alanine and lactate created from pyruvate, which can be changed over into glucose by the liver. Since quite a bit of human bulk is protein, this marvel is liable for the dying of bulk found in starvation. Be that as it may, the body can pick which cells will separate protein and which won't.

Around 2–3 g of protein must be separated to integrate 1 g of glucose; around 20–30 g of protein is separated every day to make 10 g of glucose to keep the mind alive. Be that as it may, this number may diminish the more drawn out the fasting time frame is proceeded, to preserve protein.

Starvation follows when the fat stores are totally depleted and protein is the lone fuel source accessible to the body. Subsequently, after times of starvation, the deficiency of body protein influences the capacity of significant organs, and passing outcomes, regardless of whether there are as yet fat holds left. In a more slender individual, the fat stores are drained quicker, and the protein, sooner, consequently passing happens sooner. Eventually, the reason for death is in everyday cardiovascular arrhythmia or heart failure, welcomed on by tissue debasement and electrolyte lopsided characteristics. Things like metabolic acidosis may likewise murder starving individuals.

Chapter 2. When your Body starts Burning Fats

Around 100-120 grams of glycogen can be stored in your liver, while 400-500 grams can be stored in your muscles. It will last longer when you're just sitting on the couch watching Netflix than if you're running a marathon, but in general, you'll get about an hour and a half to two hours of energy out of your stored glycogen until it's exhausted. Most people, though, never make it this far. If you eat every few hours to prevent "starvation mode" (discussed later in this chapter), you're constantly replenishing your glycogen reserves, which means you're still burning glycogen for energy.

2.1 Fat Cells in your Body

When you fast, on the other hand, you cause your glucose and glycogen stores to deplete to the point that your body is forced to search for energy elsewhere, which it does by turning to your own body fat. When your body's glucose and glycogen levels drop, it begins to break down fats in your body into glycerol and fatty acids, a process known as lipolysis. Glycerol is transported to the liver, where it undergoes gluconeogenesis. Glycerol is converted to glucose and glycogen during gluconeogenesis, which helps replenish your liver glycogen reserves. Since your brain and central nervous system depend on sugar for energy, this phase is critical. Some of the free fatty acids are transported to your muscle tissues and used as energy, while others are broken down and converted to ketones in your liver through a process known as beta-oxidation.

Many of us might be thinking about "burning some fat" so that we can look better in our bathing suits at the beach or at the pool. But what exactly does that imply?

Fat Burning Diet Chart

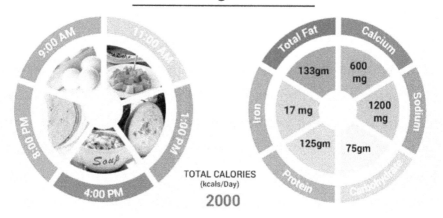

2.1.1 Function of Fat Cells

The primary function of a fat cell is to store energy. To accommodate extra energy from high-calorie foods, the body can increase the number of fat cells and their size. It can also begin to deposit fat cells on our muscles, liver, and other organs to make room for all of the extra energy from calorie-dense diets particularly when combined with a sedentary lifestyle.

Fat storage has historically served humans well. When there was no food available or a predator was pursuing us, the energy was stored as small packets of molecules called fatty acids, which were released into the bloodstream and used as fuel by muscles and other organs. In these circumstances, fat storage provided a survival advantage. Those that had a proclivity for storing fat were able to go longer stretches without eating and had more energy to deal with aggressive conditions.

When was the last time you had to flee from a predator? With an abundance of food and healthy living conditions in modern times, many people have accumulated an excess of fat stock. In fact, obesity affects more than a third of the adult population in the United States.

2.1.2 Why Fat Cells Release Less Energy

The main issue with excess fat is that the fat cells, known as adipocytes, are dysfunctional. They have an abnormally high rate of energy storage and an abnormally slow rate of energy release. Furthermore, these extra and swollen fat cells emit excessive levels of various hormones. These hormones contribute to disease by increasing inflammation, slowing metabolism, and slowing metabolism. Adiposopathy is a complex pathological mechanism of excess fat and dysfunction that makes treating obesity extremely difficult.

When someone starts and sticks to a new workout routine while still limiting calories, the body does two things to "burn fat." To begin, it taps into the energy stored in fat cells to power new operation. Second, it reduces the amount of stuff put away for storage.

Fat cells are signaled by the brain to release energy packets, or fatty acid molecules, into the bloodstream. These fatty acids are picked up by the muscles, lungs, and heart, which break them apart and use the energy contained in the bonds to carry out their functions. The scraps that remain are expelled by respiration, carbon dioxide exhaled, or urine. This makes the fat cell useless by leaving it hollow. Since the cells have a short lifetime, when they die, the body absorbs the empty cast rather than replacing it. Instead of storing energy (calories) from food, the body extracts it directly to the organs that need it over time.

As a result, the body adjusts by reducing the number and size of fat cells, improving baseline metabolism, reducing inflammation, treating illness, and extending lives. If we keep this up, the body will reabsorb the excess fat cells and discard them as waste, making us leaner and healthier on several levels.

2.2 How to lose Body Fats

To lose weight and get in shape, you must follow a healthy diet and exercise on a regular basis. The first thing you should know about exercise is that simply burning calories does not imply that you are burning fat. When you work out, the main goal should be to lose body fat, and you can't lose body fat just by burning calories.

When we exercise, our bodies continue to burn calories, but the calories consumed are those that have been accumulated as carbohydrates throughout our bodies. For your body to burn calories from stored fat, oxygen must be available. Your body requires a certain amount of oxygen to begin burning fat, and the only way to determine how much your body requires is to keep up with your target heart rate when exercising. Please keep in mind that if you just burn calories from carbohydrates, you will lose mostly "water weight," which will cause your metabolism to slow down. Consider the energy calories to be the calories you burn from carbohydrates. If you burn too many carbohydrates, your muscles won't get enough energy to boost your metabolism, which will cause fat to be burned indirectly. As a result, when you're on an exercise regimen, you'll need to up your calorie consumption to offset the energy calories you've burned.

2.2.1 What happen when you do Aerobic Exercise?

During aerobic exercise, the body goes through multiple stages before reaching the point where fat is burned. People will tell you that within the first 10 minutes of exercise, you are just burning sugar (carbohydrates) and not fat. To some degree, this is right. I say this because if you're not working out hard enough for your body to crave more oxygen, or if you're working out too hard and can't supply your body with enough oxygen for fat burning, you'll keep burning sugar after the 10-minute mark. When you exercise, keep a steady pace (not too fast, not too slow) so that your body can use stored fat as an energy source rather than carbohydrates or sugar. It's also worth noting that just because you've reached the fat-burning stage doesn't mean you'll stay there. If you are moving at a speed that is appropriate for your body, you will remain in the fat-burning stage. Check to see if the heart rate is in the target range.

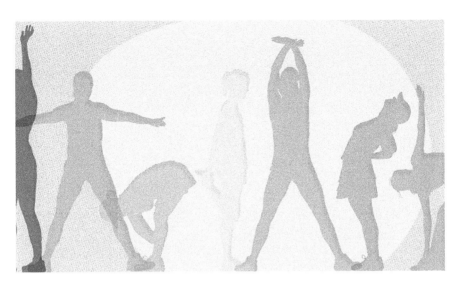

Weight training is an anaerobic workout that allows you to burn fat calories for hours after you have finished working out. Weight lifting is necessary for fat loss when at rest. Anaerobic exercise, such as weight lifting, burns more calories than aerobic exercise. The calories you burn during weight lifting workouts are mostly carbohydrate calories (which means you'll need to eat even more calories every day to maintain your energy levels), while the calories you burn during cardio workouts are mostly fat calories (which means you'll need to eat even more calories every day to maintain your energy levels) while the calories you burn at rest are mostly fat calories. Weight training boosts your metabolism, which uses your stored fat as energy, so you're burning fat even though you're not working out. You can consume fat calories if you can improve your metabolism at rest, which is difficult.

Chapter 3. Role of Ketones in Intermittent Fasting

The liver produces ketone molecules, which are water-soluble molecules. When your body does not produce enough insulin to turn glucose into energy, they are made from fatty acids.

3.1 Ketones as Alternative Source of Energy

Simply put, ketones (or ketone bodies) are an alternative fuel produced by your liver when glucose (sugar) is insufficient for energy. When your body doesn't have enough sugar or glucose to work, it needs to find a new source of energy. As a result, your body will begin to break down fat for energy. Fats are converted to a chemical called ketones in the liver during this process. The ketones, which are a form of fatty acid, are then released from the liver and enter the bloodstream, where they are used as fuel to power the body's metabolism and help muscle function.

When insulin levels are low, the body requires ketones. Fasting, low-carb diets, and sleeping overnight are all examples of when the body creates this alternative energy source.

KETONE BODIES

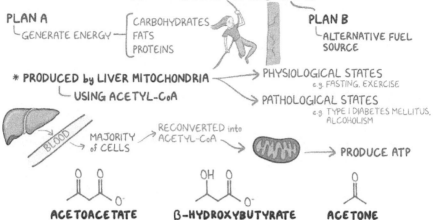

PLAN A
└ GENERATE ENERGY ─┤ CARBOHYDRATES / FATS / PROTEINS

PLAN B
└ ALTERNATIVE FUEL SOURCE

* **PRODUCED by LIVER MITOCHONDRIA**
└ USING ACETYL-CoA

→ PHYSIOLOGICAL STATES
  e.g. FASTING, EXERCISE

→ PATHOLOGICAL STATES
  e.g. TYPE I DIABETES MELLITUS, ALCOHOLISM

BLOOD → MAJORITY of CELLS → RECONVERTED into ACETYL-CoA → → PRODUCE ATP

ACETOACETATE **β-HYDROXYBUTYRATE** **ACETONE**

3.1.1 When Ketones released in body

Ketones may be released in uncontrolled type 1 diabetes due to a lack of insulin-producing beta cells in the pancreas or a lack of an exogenous, or external, insulin source. When your liver breaks down fats, it releases ketones, which are a form of chemical. When you hard, exercise for long periods of time, or don't eat as many carbohydrates, your body uses ketones for energy. Ketone levels in the blood can be poor without causing any problems.

Ketone levels in the blood, on the other hand, are a warning that something isn't quite right. Checking for ketones in your blood will tell you whether you have a lot of them. Your doctor should be able to tell you what your target range is and what you should do if you exceed it. If you're taking insulin to manage your diabetes, your body should be converting the sugar in your blood into energy.

When ketones accumulate in the bloodstream, they can become acidic, resulting in diabetic ketoacidosis (DKA). This can be life-threatening, so you should be aware of the signs and symptoms of DKA, as well as how to detect them and seek help as soon as possible.

People with type 1 diabetes are more likely to develop DKA than those with other forms of diabetes. However, if you have type 2 diabetes and take insulin, you should be on the lookout for signs of DKA.

DKA is also common among people who haven't been diagnosed with type 1 diabetes, especially children. So, if you're a parent who doesn't know anything about diabetes, this is useful information to have.

If you don't inject enough insulin or skip a dose of insulin, you're more likely to develop ketones. It's important to understand that there are occasions that you'll need more insulin and may need to monitor for elevated blood sugars more often, such as when you're not feeling good, have had an accident or operation, are pregnant, or are on your period. All of these events are common in everyday life, and they can serve as a reminder that diabetes is still present.

The normal blood ketone levels vary from one individual to the next. You're at risk of DKA if your blood ketone levels are too high. If you think you may have DKA, go to the nearest emergency room right away because you'll need hospital care. If you're not sure if you need to go to the hospital, contact your doctor or the diabetes team right away. We've got a lot of info on DKA and what you can do if your ketones are too heavy. The most important thing to keep in mind is that you should not dismiss your findings.

3.1.2 How Ketones are formed

When your body breaks down fat, ketones are formed. This means that if you have a lot of ketones in your system, you could lose weight. To lose weight, some people adopt a ketogenic diet. This is a very low carbohydrate diet that causes ketones to be produced in the blood. This is ketosis, not DKA, since there is no acidity in the blood. As ketones build up in the blood, it becomes acidic, and since there is no insulin, blood glucose levels are normally high. If you're thinking of going on a ketogenic diet, talk to your diabetes team first.

When there isn't enough sugar or glucose to meet the body's fuel needs, ketones shape. This happens in the middle of the night, as well as during dieting or fasting. Insulin levels are low during these times, but glucagon and epinephrine levels are normal. Fat is released from fat cells due to a combination of low insulin and relatively normal glucagon and epinephrine levels. Fats are transported via the bloodstream to the liver, where they are converted into ketone units. The ketone units are then reabsorbed into the bloodstream and used to power your body's metabolism by muscle and other tissues.

Ketone formation is the body's natural adaptation to malnutrition in people without diabetes. Since the production of blood sugar is controlled by a precise combination of insulin, glucagon, and other hormones, blood sugar levels never rise too high.

3.2 Intermittent Fasting and Ketosis

As well as eating a high-fat eating regimen and restricting starches, the metabolic, fat-consuming condition of ketosis can be incited by fasting. Not at all like keto, fasting isn't an eating regimen, yet rather a strategy. It doesn't figure out what you eat but instead when you eat. There are a couple of various sorts of intermittent fasting, which will change on your daily practice and timetable.

3.2.1 Eating Ketogenic Food Source

Eating ketogenic food sources can make fasting simpler on the grounds that the high fat substance causes you to feel full with less food. Fasting can assist you with getting ketosis faster, which assists you with seeing the advantages, for example, weight reduction and mental lucidity significantly earlier.

Before you start to see the unbelievable impacts of fasting ketosis, you may insight at any rate one of a few normal manifestations. While you may at first figure the eating regimen isn't working for you, this is a characteristic response, and these manifestations are just impermanent as your body is adjusting to being in ketosis.

Joined with a high fat, low carb diet, fasting can help your body consume unsaturated fats rather than glucose quicker and begin creating ketones. Following possibly 14 days you'll prepare your appetite chemicals to adjust, however before all else you may insight in any event one of the accompanying impermanent manifestations.

As food is disposed of while fasting and your body consumes its glucose, glycogen stores in the muscles are decreased. Glycogen is answerable for muscle maintenance and holds a lot of water, so as its levels fall a great deal of water is delivered. For every gram of glycogen, your body clutches three grams of water away, which can accumulate in additional pounds.

3.3 Deficiency of Water and Ketosis

Your kidneys will likewise discharge more sodium as insulin drops. This is the reason individuals who start a low carb diet or a quick regularly experience a major introductory loss of water weight and decreased swelling, before it goes to a level once glycogen stores have been completely exhausted. This weight will return when significant degrees of carbs are burned-through again and glycogen stores are topped off, which the reason is changing to a keto diet from fasting helps your body stay in ketosis.

With the deficiency of abundance water, your body additionally flushes out electrolytes like sodium, potassium and magnesium. Your body needs to create sugar for energy when fasting, so it starts an interaction called gluconeogenesis, during which your liver proselytes' non-starch materials like lactate, amino acids, and fats into glucose. As this happens, your basal metabolic rate (BMR) utilizes less energy and your circulatory strain and pulse are brought down. Consider this your body going into "power saving mode".

This can make you feel bizarrely drained and feeble until things balance out additional. This is frequently a side effect that makes individuals quit fasting before they get into ketosis and see the advantages. Recall that this progress doesn't happen quickly and you need to give your body time to change, since it's not used to going significant length of time without food. Try not to hope to be loaded with energy as you start intermittent fasting.

As your body changes with fasting and ketosis, you may encounter yearning or sugar longings two or three days. This is an ordinary response to a decrease in calorie admission, yet it likewise has to do with your chemicals. Specialists have discovered cells in the stomach, which manage the arrival of a chemical related with craving called ghrelin, are constrained by a circadian clock that is set by supper time designs. This implies that after a set number of suppers at explicit occasions every day is a prepared conduct.

When you understand this, and you're running on ketone bodies, fasting feels a lot simpler, and fasting can adjust your yearning chemicals and diminish desires for unfortunate food sources, particularly sugar and carbs. Craving side effects can likewise be set off by drying out, so make certain to remain hydrated. After changing to eating keto subsequent to fasting, following a feast plan can be useful in keeping away from yearnings and adhering to your eating regimen.

You may see terrible breath that takes on a fruity smell in the underlying phases of fasting. This is an aftereffect of raised ketone levels, specifically the ketone acetone, which is delivered through the breath. Acetone is made unexpectedly from the breakdown of acetoacetate and is the least complex and most unstable ketone. It diffuses into the lungs and ways out the body when you breathe out.

This wears off inside the primary week or something like that, yet meanwhile you could brush your teeth all the more frequently or attempt some without sugar gum. The terrible breath may likewise be joined by a dry mouth feeling. A few group may see an adjustment of solid discharges during the principal periods of ketosis. The runs or clogging may happen as changes occur in your gut's micro biome.

Stool is framed from the food that is devoured, and relying upon your individual body it can require as long as three days for food to be processed. From that point the leftover material will frame stool, after which gut motility helps push it out during crap. At the point when you're not eating food, there isn't sufficient material to shape stool: your entrails are empty. This, notwithstanding an absence of fiber admission, is the reason numerous individuals experience blockage while fasting.

3.3.1 Always be Hydrated

Different reasons could incorporate not remaining hydrated enough or affectability to certain keto food varieties. This will vary from one individual to another as each body is unique. Take psyllium husk or actuated charcoal during this stage to assist with loose bowels, and make certain to consistently drink heaps of water.

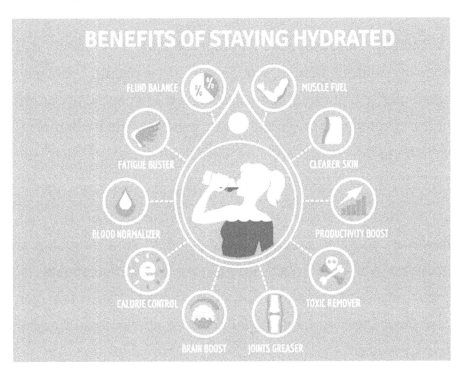

Absence of hydration can cause minor, impermanent muscle cramps in certain individuals when in fasting ketosis. Torments and hurts may likewise be brought about by malnourishment and deficient degrees of minerals supplements. Specifically, magnesium, potassium and calcium insufficiencies can cause muscle torments because of an awkwardness of electrolytes.

You may decide to renew your magnesium levels with enhancements to cure this. Attempt to build the measure of water you're drinking as a precaution alert, particularly in the primary week as drying out can be the fundamental driver of leg cramps. You can likewise keep away from espresso, a diuretic, which can additionally dry out you.

Consistent energy is an advantage of both a ketogenic diet and intermittent fasting, yet in the early phases, you may encounter a plunge in energy levels as your body adjusts to utilizing ketones for fuel. Carbs are generally the fundamental wellspring of energy and the abrupt limitation of them will normally bring about feeling depleted.

Diminished actual execution from the outset isn't exceptional, however it's just transitory. Your body is attempting to preserve however much energy as could reasonably be expected, so attempt to back off on the off chance that you can. Over the long haul you'll find more noteworthy, steadier energy levels.

An increment in pulse may occur inside the initial not many long stretches of fasting or being in ketosis. On the off chance that you regularly have lower circulatory strain, this is more probable. Heart palpitations can happen from absence of water and salt, making it essential to expand your admission of both.

3.4 Ketogenic Diet Side effects

Since a ketogenic diet can help improve circulatory strain, those on drugs that influence pulse may have to talk with their PCP about dose. When starting the keto diet, you may encounter what's normally known as the "keto influenza" as your body adjusts to fat consuming. Be that as it may, when fasting, you can really forestall or diminish the odds of keto influenza side effects, since it launches the interaction! Each time you eat, there will be some glucose delivered into the circulation system (regardless of whether it's an exceptionally limited quantity) and an insulin reaction will follow. This reaction can last as long as 20 hours, so when you quick for over 20 hours, ketones will rapidly start to supplant glucose.

While the side effects will probably be less sensational when fasting than eating a ketogenic diet, you actually may encounter the keto influenza in the initial not many long stretches of ketosis. Here are the results to know about.

On the off chance that your body isn't keto adjusted or used to fasting, you'll probably feel transient weakness toward the beginning. This is because of the electrolyte misfortune and parchedness, joined with a withdrawal from carbs and sugar as your body adjusts. Remember that it's brief, and expect to rest during and keep away from difficult actual work.

Cerebral pains are normally a consequence of drying out and electrolyte inadequacy because of bringing down blood glucose and insulin levels. This can be kept away from by appropriate hydration and electrolyte recharging through entire food sources or potentially supplements.

While you'll before long notification raised temperament levels, you may end up raging at individuals more than expected while your body changes. Crankiness isn't unprecedented during a time of withdrawal from carbs and sugar, which is just upgraded by the other keto influenza indications. Some dark espresso can give energy and liven your temperament on the off chance that you have a feeling that you need something to tame your transitory surliness.

Ketosis can prompt more mental clearness, however from the start you may wind up feeling confounded, careless or hazy. In the event that your body is utilized to a glucose exciting ride, bringing down levels can trigger cerebrum mist. It can appear regardless of how much rest you get or whether you've had espresso. Attempt to go into the principal little while of fasting monitoring the potential mind mist, as it takes some effort to progress.

A feeling of drowsiness is conceivable in the initial not many long periods of fasting. You may feel exhausted and dormant, as your glucose levels are bringing down while your body adjusts. Make certain to keep away from any potential stressors like mental strains or an absence of rest.

Much the same as the normal influenza, you may feel hot when entering ketosis. It's conceivable that in the event that you are consuming fat, that it could cause an increment in heat which prompts a raised temperature, anyway there isn't sufficient convincing proof to decide this. Since we've covered a portion of the principle concerns when fasting and entering ketosis, we should talk about how to best arrangement with them as your body changes.

While most fasting ketosis results are brief, there are a few things you can do to diminish the side effects and make the interaction more wonderful. Attempt to get sufficient rest and work on diminishing pressure however much as could reasonably be expected. When joining intermittent fasting with a ketogenic diet, ensure you're actually remaining inside your macros and eating enough calories during your eating periods.

You can expect a major flush in water weight, which can leave you dried out and fuel the above indications. Drink a lot of water and devour bone stocks that are plentiful in minerals. As your body flushes out water from absence of carbs, sodium is discharged too. For best outcomes, utilize top notch ocean salt, for example, Celtic ocean salt or Himalayan ocean salt, each time you eat.

3.4.1 How to avoid Lost Electrolytes

In case you're doing intermittent fasting, make certain to eat high-supplement dinners during your eating windows to supplant any lost electrolytes. Eat a lot of verdant greens, celery, kelp, cucumber, meat, poultry, fish, avocados and high fat, quality dairy items (if dairy concurs with you). You'll likewise need to eat a lot of fats, for example, coconut oil and MCT oil, as they'll keep you satisfied without spiking your insulin level.

Take magnesium citrate to help balance hydration and electrolyte levels. Be cautious with this on the off chance that you experience looseness of the bowels, and on the off chance that you have kidney issues, check with your primary care physician prior to taking magnesium supplements.

One approach to keep away from keto influenza manifestations is by taking exogenous ketones. They furnish your body with additional ketones to use for fuel during the progress, getting you into ketosis quicker. Accelerating the interaction can help decrease the entirety of the basic indications referenced previously.

Ensure you're dealing with yourself. Regardless of whether you're beginning another ketogenic diet, attempting intermittent fasting or both, ketosis is a change for your body. Realize you're benefiting yourself, and remember you're drawn out wellbeing if your indications baffle you. Make certain to get a lot of rest. Lack of sleep can bring down testosterone, which cause insulin opposition and make your glucose levels rise.

On the off chance that these manifestations make them feel anxious about your new keto diet, remember that there are numerous good indications of fasting in ketosis. When you get past the two or three weeks you'll be receiving the stunning rewards.

3.5 Benefits of Ketosis in Intermittent Fasting

Not exclusively does fasting in ketosis normally lessen food admission and increment fat misfortune, eating a high-fat, low carb diet likewise builds satiety and normally diminishes craving. After you overcome the underlying periods of ketosis, an incredible advantage of changing from a carb-weighty eating routine to a low-carb diet is an all the more constant flow of energy. Fasting in ketosis diminishes spikes in glucose much more, leaving you with more steady energy levels for the duration of the day.

The ketones created when consuming fat, regardless of whether you're fasting or eating a ketogenic diet, can cross the blood-cerebrum hindrance, giving energy to your mind and in any event, giving neurons protective advantages.

Other than the prompt positive indications of fasting in ketosis, there are astonishing long haul medical advantages of running on fat rather than glucose, including diminishing the danger of sicknesses like diabetes, Alzheimer's and disease.

Eating a ketogenic diet and fasting routinely can build your odds of a long, solid life. Monitoring the normal indications and utilizing the safeguard gauges above can assist you with keeping away from at first awkward results, and get the most out intermittent fasting.

Chapter 4. Intermittent Fasting versus Calories Restriction

Intermittent fasting may seem like simply an extravagant name for calorie limitation, however the two ways to deal with eating aren't something very similar. Calorie limitation includes bringing down your day by day calorie admission with an end goal to get more fit. Most calorie-confined eating regimens don't have set rules on when you can eat, yet there are typically sure food sources that are untouchable. With intermittent fasting, you limit eating to foreordained windows of time.

At the end of the day, you eat just during certain time spans. Since you have less an ideal opportunity to eat during the day, intermittent fasting may normally prompt calorie limitation, however eating less calories isn't the primary objective. In the event that weight reduction is your objective, both eating strategies will assist you with getting, however intermittent fasting has a few benefits over day by day calorie limitation.

In a survey distributed in Obesity Reviews in 2011, specialists investigated the entirety of the examinations on intermittent fasting and calorie limitation and found that while the two techniques brief a comparable measure of weight reduction, individuals will in general hold more slender bulk with intermittent fasting. At the end of the day, intermittent fasting improves your body creation, or diminish your muscle versus fat ratio, as opposed to simply bringing down the number on the scale. Different investigations show that intermittent fasting is more powerful at adjusting the appetite chemicals, ghrelin and leptin, so these sorts of diets are simpler to keep up for the long stretch. Then again, numerous ladies who depend on calorie limitation as a strategy for weight reduction wind up recovering the weight once they return to eating a typical measure of calories.

4.1 Calorie-Confined Eating

A calorie-confined eating regimen can make it simpler to get in shape and keep the pounds off. Food quality matters most, yet you actually need to watch your energy admission and adhere to your calorie objectives. The key is to ensure that your calorie admission is lower than your energy consumption.

As indicated by a generally referred to examine distributed in the diary Cell Metabolism in May 2018, cutting only 15% of your calorie admission can moderate maturing and cause critical weight reduction in just two years. Subjects who ate 15% less calories for two years dropped 17.6 pounds and encountered a significant decrease in oxidative pressure markers. As the specialists call attention to, calorie limitation diminishes energy use, prompting a more extended life.

Calorie-limited eating regimens support wellbeing and prosperity, with benefits that go past fat misfortune. At the point when you cut calories over the long haul, your body turns out to be more proficient at using energy. Fat, for example, is utilized for fuel as opposed to put away in fat tissues.

Another investigation, included in the American Journal of Clinical Nutrition in February 2017, tracked down that limiting calories by 25% more than two years can diminish fat mass and midriff circuit, increment slender weight and improve cardio metabolic wellbeing in non-hefty grown-ups.

The investigation members lost around 11% of their weight following one year and 10 percent (contrasted with their underlying body weight) following two years of calorie limitation. Men lost essentially more fat than ladies (28 versus 38 percent). These discoveries demonstrate that a calorie-confined eating regimen works with weight reduction as well as improves body piece also known as muscle-to-fat proportion.

Moreover, it might help diminish circulatory strain, glucose levels and fiery markers in individuals with diabetes, as indicated by a January 2017 clinical preliminary distributed in Diabetes. Before the finish of the examination, diabetic subjects who diminished their calorie admission had lower terrible cholesterol levels, higher great cholesterol levels and diminished pulse.

Have you ever known about the 5:2 eating routine arrangement? Shouldn't something be said about the Warrior diet? These are only two instances of calorie-confined weight control plans. Contingent upon your inclinations and how much weight you need to lose, you can likewise attempt substitute day fasting, occasional fasting or time-confined taking care of.

Any weight reduction plan that restricts your day by day calorie consumption falls into this classification. For instance, on the off chance that you typically burn-through 2,500 calories each day and, change to a 1,200-calorie diet, you're essentially confining your calorie admission. Some eating regimen plans, however, are less adaptable than others. A 500-calorie dinner plan, for instance, can influence your wellbeing and cause serious supplement inadequacies.

When all is said in done, crash abstains from food are amazingly low in calories. These weight reduction plans give just brief outcomes and may bring about kidney harm, unusual pulse, and lack of hydration and electrolyte uneven characters, as Penn Medicine calls attention to.

4.2 Advantages of Calorie Restriction

As referenced above, calorie limitation is useful. Notwithstanding, the eating routine plans utilized in clinical preliminaries are healthfully solid and share nothing practically speaking with very restricted eating regimens, for example, the cabbage soup diet, the lemonade diet or the taking care of cylinder diet.

Take the Warrior diet, for instance. This dietary example is to a great extent dependent on intermittent fasting, which means it includes times of next to zero food admission followed by times of taking care of. Weight watchers should avoid nourishment for 20 hours every day and eat inside a four-hour window around evening time. Defenders say that this is the manner by which people ate a long period of time back.

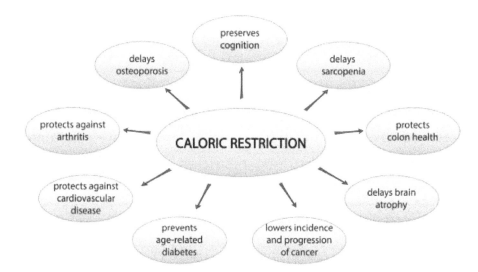

Lamentably, no investigations have been led on the Warrior diet. Nonetheless, there is a lot of proof to help the medical advantages of intermittent fasting (IF) and food limitation.

As indicated by a survey distributed in Proceedings of the Nutrition Society in August 2017, IF may trigger metabolic changes that lead to weight reduction and lessen ectopic fat, which comprises of greasy stores in or around the liver, heart, kidneys, muscles and different organs and tissues. This sort of fat has been connected to a more serious danger of aggravation, insulin obstruction, heart occasions and disabled kidney work.

Another exploration paper included in the International Journal of Obesity in December 2014 recommends that mainstream intermittent fasting conventions, for example, the 5:2 eating regimen plan, work with weight reduction by decreasing absolute food consumption. The drawback is that fasting builds hunger, so you may wind up eating more and quit consuming less calories inside and out. Day by day calorie limitation is more manageable over the long haul and may have better wellbeing results.

Regardless of whether you choose day by day calorie limitation or intermittent fasting, the way to weight reduction is to make a calorie shortage. Essentially, you need to either consume a larger number of calories than you take in or eat less calories than you consume.

As the Mayo Clinic notes, one pound of fat equivalents 3,500 calories (this number isn't unchangeable, however). This implies that in the event that you cut 3,500 calories from your day by day dinners or consume work out, you'll lose one pound.

Attempt to decide your present energy consumption. For instance, if you're eating regimen gives 2,000 calories each day that is 14,000 calories each week. To shed two pounds each week, it's important to remove 7,000 calories. In this way, you should change to a 1,000-calorie diet and plan your dinners in like manner.

Here's one stunt you can utilize: Fill up on food sources that are high in water, fiber or protein. Cucumbers, for instance, are more than 95% water and have only 8 calories for every cup, so appreciate them whenever without stressing over your weight. Protein-rich food sources, for example, turkey bosom, fish and eggs, increment satiety and may improve body synthesis, while fiber keeps you full more.

Nuts, seeds, olive oil and other supplement thick food sources are solid and brimming with flavor. The disadvantage is that they're high in calories. Pistachios, for example, brag 159 calories for every serving (1 Oz). A great many people eat significantly something other than one serving immediately, so the calories can add up rapidly.

Hoping to tack a couple of years on to the furthest limit of your life, or make the most of your brilliant years with life, great wellbeing, and energy? Examination on creatures shows a limited calorie diet may have these impacts and moderate the hands of time.

Presently, specialists of calorie limitation are trusting that people can likewise drink from the wellspring of youth. While the truth will surface eventually on the off chance that it really works, specialists and devotees say something regarding the science behind the hypothesis, and the advantages and disadvantages of a confined calorie diet.

There is considerable proof that proposes generally gentle adaptations of this eating regimen lower fasting glucose levels, which will fundamentally decrease the likelihood that an individual will get type 2 diabetes. There is also substantial evidence, albeit not as immediate, that anyone following a light version of this diet will reduce his risk of cardiovascular disease. Also, there is proof, despite the fact that it's the most un-immediate, that the likelihood of somebody on a confined calorie diet getting malignant growth goes down.

4.3 Disadvantages of Calories Restriction

While calorie limitation is a compelling method to get more fit at first, keeping up that weight reduction is another story. Studies show that supported calorie shortfalls or confining your calorie admission for a significant stretch of time can build the strength and recurrence of food longings in ladies and increment the craving to utilize food as a prize. Diminishing calorie admission triggers hormonal changes that increment your craving, decline your metabolic rate, and make you need to eat unhealthy food sources. Here are the principle chemicals that are contrarily influenced by calorie limitation:

• Leptin

• Peptide YY

• Cholecystokinin

• Insulin

- Ghrelin

- Gastric inhibitory polypeptide

- Pancreatic polypeptide

Much seriously disrupting that these negative hormonal changes can endure for longer than a year even after you quit consuming less calories, as indicated by research distributed in Perspectives on Psychological Science in 2017. That is the reason when you center just on limiting calories, you feel hungry constantly and struggle zeroing in on anything besides food. Your chemicals are so messed up that they're continually advising your body you need to eat, regardless of whether you just had a supper. Since your digestion is additionally easing back down, you'll need to keep dropping your day by day calorie admission to keep getting results. One-to 66% of individuals who limit calories as a way to weight reduction recover all the weight, yet they likewise recapture significantly more weight than they lost in any case!

4.3.1 Calories Count must be Checked Carefully

While the effortlessness of checking calories causes this way to deal with appear to be simple, sadly, there is something else entirely to food than just calories. Picking your food decisions exclusively dependent on numbers may diminish the calories you devour, however on the off chance that you are eating a predominately low calorie shoddy nourishment diet, the weight may fall off, yet it very well may be to the detriment of your wellbeing. A low calorie diet isn't consequently a solid eating routine. While some orange soft drink contains less calories than a similar measure of squeezed orange, the soft drink can't compare to the juice with regards to nourishment. Soft drink is essentially sugar disintegrated in water and without some other supplements. In examination, eight ounces of OJ will meet your nutrient C requirements for the afternoon and is likewise a brilliant wellspring of potassium. To refreshingly get in shape, you ought to follow a lower calorie, even eating regimen that meets your wholesome requirements by giving an assortment of food sources, like entire grains, natural products, vegetables, fish, lean meats, poultry, dairy, and some vegetable oils.

Another alert about low calorie consumes less calories is that in the event that you become excessively fanatical about calorie tallying and decrease your calories excessively low, you could be putting yourself in danger of passing up significant supplements, like calcium and iron? It can turn out to be amazingly trying for ladies to meet their everyday supplement needs on the off chance that they are burning-through under 1,600 calories day by day.

Burning-through a low calorie diet can likewise cause weight reduction to happen too quickly and may cause you to feel exhausted and sick, cause clogging, and can likewise propagate the development of gallstones. While getting in shape at a pace of roughly half to 2 pounds week after week is for the most part viewed as protected, a more reasonable objective is lose around 10% of your body weight over a six-month time frame. At the end of the day, in the event that you are overweight and need to shed 18 pounds, put your focus on losing close to 3 pounds per month or not exactly a pound seven days throughout the following a half year.

Before you embrace a low-calorie diet, it's fundamental to be careful about the expected dangers. The main threat of limiting your calories is just trying too hard. While eating somewhat less than expected can help your wellbeing and prosperity, going excessively far can hurt your wellbeing differently.

Calorie limitation can likewise influence you intellectually. The glucose you lose when you eat too little can make you feel intellectually lazy and conceivably lead to memory issues. In case you're experiencing difficulty thinking, this may likewise be a side effect of under eating.

Ceaselessly following calories can be dreary, particularly on the off chance that you have a bustling way of life or eat on the run. Confining calories may likewise cause a few group to feel on edge and surprisingly masochist about devouring excessively.

Calorie including may bring about forsaking the eating routine or building up a dietary problem due to being exorbitantly cautious about the quantity of calories devoured. How would you get more fit and afterward keep up your optimal weight in the event that you don't check calories? Figure out how to eat the perfect measure of solid, entire food varieties, and consolidate it with exercise and stress decrease.

The calories from the food varieties you eat are prepared in an unexpected way, contingent upon the food varieties you eat. Calories from supplement thick food varieties like spinach, chicken, eggs, new products of the soil took care of meat top you off and keep you full for quite a while, causing you to eat less. Fiber from vegetables, nuts, entire grains and other quality food sources are more earnestly for your body to separate and process. Eating these sorts of food varieties power your body to consume fat.

You're bound to indulge sweets, inexpensive food burgers, cake, fries and other handled food since they don't top you off as quick. Rather than causing your body to consume fat, these food varieties urge your body to store fat.

Chilliness, relentless craving, shortcoming, depletion, dazedness, muscle squandering, and balding were a portion of the manifestations. Heart volume shrank by 20%. Pulse eased back. Internal heat level dropped.

Resting metabolic rate dropped by 40%. Strangely, this isn't that distant from a past report from 1917 that showed Total Energy Expenditure (TEE) diminished by 30%. At the end of the day, the body was closing down. We should reconsider this from the body's perspective. The body is familiar with getting 3,200 calories each day and now it gets 1,560. To protect itself, it executes no matter how you look at it decreases in energy.

The way to recall, however, is that this guarantees endurance of the person during a period of outrageous pressure. No doubt, you may feel junky, however you'll live to tell the story. This is the savvy thing for the body to do. It isn't so moronic as to continue to consume energy it doesn't have.

Think about the other option. The body is utilized to 3,200 calories each day and now gets 1,560. The body actually consumes 3,200 calories. Things feel typical. A quarter of a year later, you are dead. It is totally incomprehensible that the body doesn't respond to caloric decrease by lessening caloric consumption.

Consider numerous assertions such that on the off chance that you lessen 500 calories each day, you will lose one pound in multi week. Does that imply that in 200 weeks you will gauge nothing? Plainly sooner or later, the body must, must, should diminish caloric use. Incidentally, the variation happens very quickly and perseveres in the long haul. More about this later.

Fanatical contemplations of food. Gorge conduct. Outrageous despondency. Extreme passionate misery. Peevishness. Loss of charisma. Interest in everything other than food disappeared. Social withdrawal and segregation. A few subjects turned out to be, in all honesty, hypochondriac. One patient apparently cut away 3 fingers with a hatchet in a demonstration of self-mutilation. In any case, I'm certain you are starting to get the image.

Consider the last time you attempted to slim down by diminishing calories and segment size. What befell their weight after the semi-starvation time frame? Along the x-hub we have the 24 weeks of the starvation time frame. Both body weight and muscle versus fat dropped. As they began upon the recuperation time frame, they recaptured the weight. As a matter of fact, the weight was recovered rather rapidly in around 12 or so weeks, the weight has returned to benchmark.

You can see that the body weight keeps on expanding until it is really higher than it was before the examination begun. Furthermore, simply see that muscle versus fat! It goes taking off above pattern. Sound recognizable? Thought so.

We should survey what happens when you go on a calorie limited, high sugar, low-fat eating regimen of 1,560 calories/day actually like your PCP or dietician right now advises you to do. You feel junky, worn out, chilly, eager, touchy, and discouraged. That is not on the grounds that you are eating less junk food, there are physiological reasons why you feel so horrible. Metabolic rate drops, chemicals make you hungry, internal heat level drops, and there are a large number of mental impacts. The most exceedingly awful thing is that you lose a touch of weight however you restore it all when the eating routine stops.

It is progressively certain that one of the critical suppositions of the Caloric Reduction as Primary hypothesis is wrong. Nonetheless, you can't, from this condition, say that lessening 'Calories In' brings about Fat Loss unless 'Calories Out' stays stable. This expects to be that 'Calories In' is totally autonomous of 'Calories Out'. This is not true. The caloric consumptions and caloric admission are inseparably connected to one another.

Said another way decreasing Calories In lessens Calories Out. Diminishing caloric admission unavoidably prompts decreased caloric use. That is the reason regular counting calories as far as we might be concerned doesn't work. I know it. You know it.

As a matter of fact, we have realized that this will generally be valid since 1917. Truth be told, in our true inner being, we most likely have consistently realized that it will generally be valid. Eating less for a drawn out period makes you drained and hungry. What's more, to top it all off... you recover all the weight you have lost. Weight lost is muscle and fat. Weight recaptured is all fat.

We have recently decided to fail to remember this badly designed certainty in light of the fact that our PCPs, our dietitians, our administration, our researchers, our government officials, and our media have all been shouting at us for quite a long time that it is about 'Calories In versus Calories Out'. Caloric Reduction is Primary. Eat less, move more, and that sort of ineptitude.

We need to totally reevaluate our customary perspective on weight. In an analysis, 18 large and 23 non-hefty subjects with a steady weight were enlisted. They were taken care of a fluid eating routine of 45% starch, 40% fat, and 15% protein until the ideal weight reduction or weight acquire was accomplished.

One gathering focused on a 10% weight reduction and the other gathering focused on a 10% weight acquire. After weight acquire, subjects were then gotten back to their underlying weight, and afterward a further 10% or 20% weight reduction was accomplished.

The inquiry they needed to answer was what ended up teeing when weight was expanded or diminished. This was accomplished without an adjustment of the arrangement of the eating regimen. That is, the fluid eating routine was a consistent proportion of starches, fats, and protein. The lone variable was the complete admission of this fluid eating routine. What ends up teeing when caloric admission is changed?

4.3.2 Caloric Reduction as Primary (CRaP) theory

All in all, on the off chance that we decrease or increment our Calories In, what befalls Calories Out? As indicated by the customary Caloric Reduction as Primary (CRaP) theory, as Calories In go up or down, there ought to be very little change in the Calories Out.

What was the deal? In the 10% weight acquire bunch, individuals expanded their energy consumption by just about 500 calories/day. Recollect that one of the critical suppositions of the CRaP hypothesis is that in light of caloric change, TEE doesn't change. This is plainly not true.

Rather than a straightforward calories in, calories out model where fat is saved by an unnecessary admission of calories, apparently the body reacts to abundance calories by attempting to consume them off! Presently how about we see what occurs as the weight is gotten back to business as usual. Here, things begin to get truly intriguing. As weight gets back to business as usual, TEE gets back to gauge. As we move into 10% and 20% weight reduction, the body lessens TEE by around 300 or 400 calories each day.

Thus, as we get thinner, the body reacts to the weight reduction by decreasing TEE. This eases back weight reduction, and empowers weight recover regardless of full consistence with the eating routine. All in all, an increment in Calories In causes an expansion in Calories Out. A reduction of Calories In causes an abatement in Calories Out. This is the body's ordinary reaction. Weight reduction will level, however not on the grounds that you weren't following the eating routine. Since that is the normal physiological reaction. It happens to everyone!

On the off chance that you were attempting to get more fit by eating less (Caloric Reduction as Primary), this is the place where you go, "Where's my sad demeanor emoticon?" Our body acts substantially more like an indoor regulator. That is, the body appears to have a specific Body Set Weight (BSW). Any endeavors to increment over this BSW will bring about our body attempting to get back to its unique load by expanding TEE (expanding digestion to consume off the abundance calories).

Any endeavors to diminish underneath this BSW will bring about our body attempting to get back to its unique load by diminishing TEE (diminishing digestion to recapture lost calories). No big surprise it is so difficult to keep the load off! As we moderate our digestion, we should further a lot diminish our caloric admission to keep up weight reduction.

Here's the confused dietary method of segment control or Caloric Restriction as Primary. We lessen our bit size yet keep feast timing and arrangement the equivalent. We decrease our calorie utilization from 2000 cal/day to 1,600 cal/day. Our weight may lessen, yet then the body would react by diminishing TEE to around 1,600 cal/day. We may feel chilly, worn out, hopeless, and hungry. On the off chance that you have ever experienced an eating regimen you most likely skill that feels.

The most exceedingly terrible piece of it is that we don't lose any further weight since we are eating less and consuming less. Any slip in the eating regimen, even to the past ordinary 2,000 cal/day will bring about weight recapture. Demoralization sets in. We become weary of feeling so horrible so we return to our normal eating regimen. All the weight returns dashing with some extra just in case.

We feel that we have bombed ourselves. We feel that it is our flaw. Our primary care physicians, dietitians, and other clinical experts quietly scrutinize us for 'fizzling'. Others quietly accept we have no 'resolution', and offer insignificant sayings. Sound natural? No doubt, I suspected as much.

In any case, in truth, the faltering was not our own. The part control diet is practically ensured to fall flat. It has been demonstrated again and again over the most recent 100 years. The solitary explanation we imagine that it works is on the grounds that everyone the specialists, the dietitians, the 'researchers', the media have persuaded us that it is about calories. No, the weak is with our wholesome specialists.

Chapter 5. Intermittent Fasting Helps Control your Hunger

A few group have extraordinary accomplishment with intermittent fasting (IF) on the grounds that fasting checks their craving. The outcome is that it assists them with adhering to it and improve its advantages. In any case, individuals vary significantly in their capacity to endure fasting so it's basic to focus on your body's reactions and what it is advising you.

During the progress from took care of fasting, an arrival of stress chemicals and an adjustment of digestion can kick in. A result is that chemicals controlling yearning and satiety can escape balance, driving us to get inert to signals that we're full when eating once more.

These changes in hunger chemicals could conceivably happen contingent upon the complete part of time you are fasting, you're eating routine and how you're executing intermittent fasting. Here, we audit the proof in regards to intermittent fasting and craving chemicals, investigate how intermittent fasting influences craving and furnish you with a couple of tips to help facilitate the change and beat hunger.

This article is definitely not a worldwide contention against intermittent fasting. Maybe, it calls attention to that the individuals who are simply beginning to quick could experience difficulty. Purportedly, the hardest piece of fasting is the principal day, and that is normally just on the off chance that you eat high-carb and additionally not used to go significant stretches without eating.

There are a few sorts of intermittent fasting. The sort most often utilized in logical examinations is substitute day intermittent fasting (ADF), while the sorts being utilized in general society are for the most part either 1-2 week by week fasting days or part day diets, similar to the 16:8 quick.

To the extent the best in class goes, there are a couple of studies on ADF, a couple on intermittent fasting suggestive of 5:2 fasting and an exceptionally predetermined number on part-day fasting (for example 16:8) following changes in hunger chemicals, at the hour of composing.

ADF likewise includes calorie restriction (CR). There are contrasts among CR and intermittent fasting where appetite and chemicals are concerned and it tends to be difficult to figure out which of the fasting or CR is affecting yearning chemicals.

In this article, the expression "fasting" will be utilized by and large to allude to the entirety of the previously mentioned intermittent fasting strategies, with explicit depiction of conventions when proper. The vast majority don't understand that there are a plenty of chemicals controlling craving, hunger and fulfillment after a feast.

Their levels and signals change with changing food admission and how much fat you're conveying. There is likewise some sign of a sexual orientation contrast in light of them. These chemicals, delivered from different organs and tissues, effects hunger and effect how well or how inadequately taking care of is directed in the mind.

5.1 Role of Leptin

Among those straightforwardly engaged with craving guideline that assume a significant part are two exceptionally compelling to the present conversation: the gut-inferred chemical ghrelin and another discharged from fat cells known as leptin.

Ghrelin invigorates craving, advances fat stockpiling and brings down energy consumption while leptin diminishes hunger, conveys a message to your cerebrum that you're full and turns eating 'off'.

Ghrelin gets entrained to typical eating times and once one beginnings fasting, its levels and discharge may change, as proposed by research from the University of Birmingham on ghrelin and taking care of recurrence. The examination contrasted a quick and a low-recurrence feast routine (two suppers) or high-recurrence one (12 little dinners) across eight hours.

The expanded feast recurrence would in general keep up stable ghrelin levels during the day and the lower dinner recurrence caused higher varieties in ghrelin. During the quick, but short, ghrelin rose marginally with time and took more time to diminish.

Amazingly, with a more extended fasting window of 24 hours, ghrelin doesn't appear to get any higher. Nonetheless, following two months of ADF, it's an alternate story. One investigation tracked down a critical expansion in ghrelin levels, even with no adjustment of genuine craving sentiments.

It has been said that constantly raised degrees of ghrelin are related with changes in muscle to fat ratio. Further exploration connected high ghrelin to positive input circles in the cerebrum's prize hardware and enthusiastic eating. No doubt, however, that issues with high ghrelin can be in any event somewhat moderated by eating an eating routine containing the correct equilibrium of supplements.

The creation of the supper that breaks the quick appears to issue to keep ghrelin levels in balance. Ghrelin is least influenced by fats, while carbs frequently cause a bounce back hyper secretion in ghrelin.

Expanding protein particularly is one approach to restrict hunger and may even keep up satiety despite high ghrelin. Ghrelin is additionally higher when sodium admission is low, so keeping a decent salt admission could have an effect. Leptin is an expert chemical with downstream impacts on different chemicals identified with hunger. A drop in leptin expands hunger and is thought to cause weight reduction levels.

Individuals who are overweight or stout ordinarily have high leptin yet are impervious to it while less fatty people may have lower levels however higher affectability. As leptin imparts signs to the cerebrum that directs satiety, an absence of leptin implies the mind will not really register fulfillment and craving could stay raised.

Expanded times of fasting perpetually lead to a misfortune in muscle to fat ratio. When this occurs, the quantity of processing plants for leptin creation (recall leptin is gotten from fat cells) will diminish, and thusly so will the supreme measure of leptin available for use.

5.1.1 Significance of Leptin Levels in Body

As indicated by research, leptin levels can quickly decrease in the abstained state and one potential aftereffect of this is an increment in craving. One examination inspecting leptin's job in weight reduction has likewise tracked down that this quick fall in light of fasting may push individuals toward gorging.

The extent of the decline in leptin changes. A transient report found that school ladies at the University of Virginia who abstained for two days encountered a 75 percent drop in leptin, albeit this was presumably remunerated by a major lift during feeding.

Another testing stout members, which included two months of ADF, found that leptin fixations were diminished by 21% before the finish of the examination. There's likewise opposing proof. Ladies fasting during Ramadan really show a major expansion in leptin. The fasting additionally diminishes neuropeptide-Y, a chemical that animates hunger.

It merits referencing that the examination neglected to address impacts of late evening eating on the body's common circadian musicality to hunger, which is intrinsic in our hereditary cosmetics and influences both leptin and ghrelin autonomously of the eat/quick cycle.

To the extent leptin goes, apparently the normal current way of life (cheap food, almost no activity, a lot pressure and insufficient rest) incredibly adds to its disturbance, with absence of rest being a significant offender.

By and large, was related with moderately more significant levels of the chemical. Interestingly, getting less rest implied lower levels of leptin and higher weight files in the investigation. So rest the suggested 8 hours every day if conceivable. If not, rest more overall as your body makes less leptin in the event that you don't get sufficient rest. In the event that you've at any point felt hungrier the day following a helpless night's rest, this could be on the grounds that your leptin levels have dropped.

Yearning isn't as straightforward as 'the more you don't eat, the more eager you'll be'. There are a lot more unpretentious sources of info and a complex hormonal guideline of appetite is having an effect on everything.

Chemicals that trigger eating, similar to ghrelin, may get enhanced because of fasting. In any case, ghrelin normally tops at day 1-2 and afterward consistently falls. This lines up with what is seen clinically, where craving is the most noticeably terrible issue at beginning. Numerous individuals on longer diets report that hunger commonly vanishes after day 2.

Fasting can likewise smother chemicals prompting satiety, as leptin, yet presumably more so if calories are confined during the eating window and when driving an undesirable way of life or not resting soundly.

Fasting impacts everybody distinctively and the negatives concerning craving guideline are more probable in slender and dynamic people, those with high feelings of anxiety and helpless dietary patterns or with conventions that take fasting to the limit.

One populace that presumably shouldn't utilize intermittent fasting are those with a past dietary problem, similar to bulimia or anorexia, or even those with a propensity towards confused eating designs.

In the present circumstance, intermittent fasting could put them directly back into the kind of exchanged limitation and gorge cycles that they had in any case and cause them to lose all out food control when fasting. Individuals who are seriously underweight, pregnant or breastfeeding ladies, and kids and young people should likewise not quick. Furthermore, anybody on prescriptions should check with their primary care physician that these are not contraindicated.

Likewise with all things, certain people might be more helpless than others to the deficiency of authority over food admission when breaking the quick. Yet, it appears to be in general more genuine for those endeavoring to restrict themselves to a solitary dinner.

For a great many people, a moderate way to deal with intermittent fasting like the 16:8 strategy, can pass on the advantages of fasting (fat consuming and insulin affectability) without altogether influencing hunger chemicals or causing uncontrolled eating.

At last, getting mindful of the feelings behind eating and making the differentiation between an indulgent drive to eat, i.e., being keen on food and exhausted, and genuine craving can make the change to fasting simpler.

ADF doesn't instigate hyperplasia (excessive eating or a strangely extraordinary craving for food) and, now and again, individual's burn-through five percent not exactly their ordinary day by day caloric admission. An examination survey of ten investigations on intermittent fasting and distraction with food discovered four didn't show expanded hunger while six showed an unbiased impact with no compensatory indulging.

5.2 What is Leptin Resistance?

Numerous individuals accept that weight gain and misfortune is about calories and resolution. Be that as it may, current corpulence research opposes this idea. Researchers progressively say that a chemical called leptin is included.

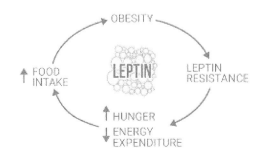

Leptin obstruction, in which your body doesn't react to this chemical, is currently accepted to be the main driver of fat addition in people. This heading discloses all you require to think about leptin and how it is involved in corpulence. Leptin is a chemical that is created by your muscle versus fat's cells.

It is frequently alluded to as the "satiety chemical" or the "starvation chemical." Leptin's essential objective is in the mind especially a territory called the nerve center. Leptin should tell your cerebrum that when you have sufficient fat put away you don't have to eat and can consume calories at an ordinary rate.

It likewise has numerous different capacities identified with richness, invulnerability and cerebrum work. Notwithstanding, leptin's fundamental job is long haul guideline of energy, including the quantity of calories you eat and consume, just as how much fat you store in your body.

The leptin framework advanced to hold people back from starving or gorging, the two of which would have made you more averse to get by in the indigenous habitat. Today, leptin is viable at holding us back from starving. Yet, something is broken in the component that should keep us from gorging.

Leptin is created by your muscle versus fat's cells. The more muscle versus fat they convey, the more leptin they produce. Leptin is conveyed by the circulation system into your mind, where it conveys a message to the nerve center the part that controls when and the amount you eat.

The fat cells use leptin to tell your mind how much muscle to fat ratio they convey. Undeniable degrees of leptin tell your cerebrum that you have a lot of fat put away, while low levels tell your mind that fat stores are low and that you need to eat.

At the point when you eat, your muscle versus fat goes up, driving your leptin levels to go up. Alternately, when you don't eat, your muscle to fat ratio goes down, driving your leptin levels to drop. This sort of framework is known as a negative input circle and like the control systems for various physiological capacities, like breathing, internal heat level and pulse. Individuals who are hefty have a ton of muscle versus fat in their fat cells.

Since fat cells produce leptin in relation to their size, individuals who are large additionally have extremely significant degrees of leptin. Given the way leptin work, numerous stout individuals ought as far as possible their food consumption. As such, their cerebrums should realize that they have a lot of energy put away.

Notwithstanding, their leptin flagging may not work. While bountiful leptin might be available, the cerebrum doesn't see it. This condition known as leptin opposition is currently accepted to be one of the principle organic supporters of corpulence.

At the point when your mind doesn't get the leptin signal, it wrongly imagines that your body is starving despite the fact that it has a sizable amount of energy put away. This makes your cerebrum change its conduct to recapture muscle to fat ratio. Your cerebrum at that point energizes:

Eating more: Your cerebrum imagines that you should eat to forestall starvation.

Diminished energy use: with an end goal to preserve energy, your mind diminishes you energy levels and causes you to consume less calories very still.

In this manner, eating more and practicing less isn't the basic reason for weight acquire but instead a potential result of leptin obstruction, a hormonal deformity. For a great many people who battle with leptin opposition, willing yourself to beat the leptin-driven starvation signal is close to unthinkable.

Leptin opposition might be one explanation that numerous eating regimens neglect to advance long haul weight reduction. In case you're leptin-safe, shedding pounds actually decreases fat mass, which prompts a huge decrease in leptin levels yet your cerebrum doesn't really switch its leptin opposition.

When leptin goes down, this prompts hunger, expanded craving, and diminished inspiration to practice and a diminished number of calories consumed very still. Your cerebrum at that point believes that you are starving and starts different amazing systems to recover that lost muscle to fat ratio.

This could be a principle motivation behind why such countless individuals yo-yo diet losing a lot of weight just to recover it presently. A few possible systems behind leptin opposition have been recognized. These include:

Aggravation: Inflammatory motioning in your nerve center is likely a significant reason for leptin obstruction in the two creatures and people.

Free unsaturated fats: Having raised free unsaturated fats in your circulation system may build fat metabolites in your mind and meddle with leptin flagging.

Having high leptin: Having raised degrees of leptin in any case appears to cause leptin obstruction.

A large portion of these components are enhanced by corpulence, implying that you could get caught in an endless loop of putting on weight and turning out to be progressively leptin safe over the long haul. The most ideal approach to know whether you are leptin safe is to glance in the mirror.

On the off chance that you have a ton of muscle to fat ratio, particularly in the gut region, at that point you are very likely leptin safe. It isn't completely clear how leptin obstruction can be switched, however hypotheses proliferate.

A few analysts accept that lessening diet-initiated aggravation may help invert leptin obstruction. Zeroing in on an in general sound way of life is additionally prone to be a successful methodology. All you have to do is:

Stay away from prepared food: Highly handled food varieties may bargain the uprightness of your gut and drive aggravation.

Eat solvent fiber: Eating dissolvable fiber can help improve your gut wellbeing and may ensure against weight.

Exercise: Physical movement may help turn around leptin opposition.

Rest: Poor rest is ensnared in issues with leptin.

Lower your fatty oils: Having high fatty substances can forestall the vehicle of leptin from your blood to your cerebrum. The most ideal approach to bring down fatty substances is to diminish your carb consumption.

Eat a lot of protein: Eating a lot of protein will lead to programmed weight loss, which may be due to an increase in leptin affectability In spite of the fact that there is no basic method to dispense with leptin obstruction, you can make long haul way of life changes that may improve your personal satisfaction.

Leptin obstruction might be one of the fundamental reasons individuals put on weight and struggle losing it. Accordingly, corpulence is normally not brought about by ravenousness, sluggishness or an absence of self-discipline.

Maybe, there are solid biochemical and social powers influencing everything too. The Western eating routine specifically might be a main driver of weight. In case you're concerned you might be impervious to leptin, there are a few stages you can take to carry on with a better way of life and conceivably improve or switch your obstruction.

5.2.1 How Intermittent Fasting Helps Improve Leptin Resistance

In our mind there is a region known as the nerve center. It primary job is homeostasis. It capacities to control our hunger, temperature, pulse, circulatory strain, liquid and electrolyte equilibrium and rest cycles. It gets data from all pieces of our sensory system and reacts by delivering chemicals. These chemicals are delivered onto our pituitary organ which creates more chemicals focused to our organs. Together, these two spaces of the cerebrum control our kidneys, adrenal organs, sex organs, bones, muscles, thyroid organ, capacity to climax and interface with our friends and family, just as produce milk after birth.

In this heading we investigate how craving and body weight are constrained by the chemical leptin and how fasting can deal with assistance manage this cycle.

Leptin is a chemical delivered by fat cells. Its capacity is to tell the mind how much fat we have with the goal that it can direct energy creation. At the point when we have sufficient fat put away, we don't have to eat to have enough calories to run the framework. Our bodies are a perplexing harmony between the measure of energy we need, the calories needed to eat and exhaust and how much fat we will store on our bodies to address that issue. It is a progressing count. The leptin framework developed so we wouldn't starve to death and now we sure aren't. Truth be told we are eating ourselves to death. Why would that be?

Leptin conveys to the mind how much fat is being conveyed with an end goal to adjust the energy/energy in necessity. Since leptin is delivered by our fat cells, when there is heaps of fat, there is bunches of leptin. In a condition of sufficient fat stores, a satiety signal is delivered in the cerebrum restraining us from devouring more calories. In low fat expresses our mind is told we are risking starvation and to increment caloric admission. This is a negative input cycle where within the sight of satisfactory fat stores, the longing to burn-through more calories is killed.

At the point when individuals are hefty, they have a great deal of fat cells and hence a ton of leptin. This over creation of leptin, combined with the over creation insulin found in heftiness, causes a leptin opposition in the mind. The cerebrum turns out to be less delicate to the signs from leptin advising it there are satisfactory fat stores. Leptin obstruction because of undeniable degrees of insulin and coursing leptin is the principle physiological instrument behind corpulence. This leptin opposition the mind signals us to both eat more, and exhaust less energy!

In spite of the fact that shedding pounds, and thusly quick cells and leptin would appear to be a smart thought, indeed it triggers the longing to eat more. At the point when we lose fat cells and leptin, we don't consequently recover leptin affectability in the mind. The decrease in circling leptin trigger a starvation impacts on the cerebrum bringing about expanded craving and diminished energy consumption.

Shedding pounds isn't the solitary aim of leptin inadequacy. There are hereditary deformities that lead to low degrees of leptin. It is assessed that roughly 3% of hefty people have a receptor deformity causing stoutness. In the United States, that is generally 2.3 million individuals.

Aggravation in the hypothalamic area of the mind has been appeared to cause leptin obstruction. Leptin has a job in managing the invulnerable framework due to its closeness fit as a fiddle and capacity to another provocative middle person called interleukin-6. The presence of the fiery marker CRP has been related with leptin opposition in corpulent people.

Different reasons for leptin opposition are because of intracellular concealment of leptin motioning just as extracellular restricting of leptin, making it inaccessible to the cells. Insulin affectability can be improved numerous ways:

diminished glucose admission, fasting, eating food varieties that help insulin affectability in cells.

5.2.2 Types of Food source and Leptin Resistance

Most of irritation in the framework comes from the gut. Explicitly eating provocative food sources, for example, handled food sources, refined sugar, GMOs, non-natural food sources, and allergenic food sources like wheat, dairy, corn and soy. Keeping away from fiery food varieties diminishes aggravation in the gut. At the point when the gut is presented to irritation throughout some undefined time frame, the tight intersections between the gut cells gets porous. Which means undigested food particles escape into the circulation system. These food particles trigger the resistant framework to create immunoglobulin against them, thinking they are unfamiliar trespassers. This cycle makes food hypersensitivities and sensitivities. The food sources we are hypersensitive to contrast individual to individual, so having them surveyed by a doctor is the initial step to aiding fix the gut. Alternate approaches to fix the gut coating and diminishing aggravation are taking enhancements demonstrated to help: fish oil, and probiotics.

Getting sufficient rest plus practicing have been appeared to bring down gut aggravation.

Exercise doesn't need to be distressing. Indeed, even 30 minutes daily has been demonstrated to bring down coronary illness and forestall diabetes. In the event that you are gazing exercise interestingly, you can utilize my brief principle.

This is essentially a stroll around a couple of squares. Getting outside likewise improves emotional well-being. Sun openness and nitrogen admission are totally related with better mind-sets. View another science called "woods washing".

Fasting, regardless of whether it is genuine water fasting or irregular is an extraordinary method to expand leptin and glucose affectability in the cells. Discontinuous fasting is the act of have 1 day of diminished calories each week or 1 complete fasting day of the week or a 16 hour quick every evening. Any of these alternatives work a similar way: allowing the body to go through the glucose and being to go through the glycogen or glucose stores. In doing this, we train our body to react less to the sign that glucose is no more. Since it knows there is another save (glycogen). What this resembles is an abatement in desperation for a bite or glucose fix. Also, it is liberating. Whatever your requirements are during the week for work, doing action or everyday life, there is a discontinuous fasting convention that meets your requirements.

Water fasting is a more concentrated type of resetting the glucose resistance and insulin affectability in cells. It includes ingesting just water for a while. By doing this, our body goes through all the glucose and glycogen energy stores and starts a cycle called Ketosis - separating fats for fuel. For more data on the most proficient method to water quick or discontinuous quick, contact our center for customized projects and guidance.

MIC represents methionine, inositol and choline and they are known as lipotropic or " fat processing". These infusions focus on the essential greasy stores in the stomach, gluteus district, hips, and internal thighs and under arms. They are a unique recipe of nutrients, supplements and cofactors intended to help the liver to breakdown and take out fats from the body.

Methionine is a fundamental amino corrosive implying that we need to eat it to have it. It aids the separate of fat in the liver which brings down your body's cholesterol and eliminates it from the circulatory framework.

The inositol part is associated with the natural motioning of fat digestion. It diminishes serum cholesterol, by advancing fat digestion. Choline is a fundamental supplement needed for the vehicle of fats and cholesterol. After separate, fats are

111

shipped to the liver where they are separated in to their segment parts and discharged from your body through bile.

Different supplements in the recipe are Vitamin B12, B-Complex and Carnitine. B nutrients are universal aides in the body's biochemical cycles. Carnitine is an amino corrosive supportive in separating fat and protecting muscle and moving fat from high thickness regions to the liver.

Through diet, individuals might be lacking in any of these supplements making fat consuming more troublesome. A normal timetable of MIC infusions can uphold the body with the supplements it needs to work appropriately as a feature of a fasting or clinical program.

Conclusion

In this book you have read about the detail mechanism of action of intermittent fasting diet plan and its stages like fed, post-absorptive and starvation. You have also read about how to burn your body fats by using intermittent fasting diet plans. After reading this book, now you are also able to know that how important is to calculate calories according to each individual specific body needs and condition and also its benefits and side effects. We have discussed about keto foods, ketosis and ketones and their importance in intermittent fasting and also how intermittent fasting diet plan helps to control your hunger and the role of leptin in it.

INTERMITTENT FASTING DIET

The complete guide on How to Make Intermittent Fasting a Lifestyle that can Weight Loss and to have Better Health.

Chapter 1. Intermittent Fasting: A Potential Diet Plan for Successful Brain Aging

The weakness of the sensory system to propelling age is very regularly show in neurodegenerative issues like Alzheimer's and Parkinson's illnesses. In this survey article we depict proof recommending that two dietary intercessions, caloric limitation (CR) and intermittent fasting (IF), can draw out the wellbeing range of the sensory system by impinging upon major metabolic and cell flagging pathways that manage life-length. CR and IF influence energy and oxygen extremist digestion, and cell stress reaction frameworks, in manners that secure neurons against hereditary and natural components to which they would somehow or another capitulate during maturing. There are numerous intelligent pathways and sub-atomic systems by which CR and IF advantage neurons including those including insulin-like flagging, FoxO record factors, sirtuins and peroxisome proliferator-initiated receptors. These pathways invigorate the creation of protein chaperones, neurotrophic elements and cancer prevention agent chemicals, all of which help cells adapt to pressure and oppose illness. A superior comprehension of the effect of CR and IF on the maturing sensory system will probably prompt novel methodologies for forestalling and treating neurodegenerative problems.

1.1 Introduction

Mind issues of maturing have as of late become driving reasons for handicap and passing, because of various advances in the anticipation and therapy of cardiovascular sickness and tumors. A few noticeable danger factors for significant age-related illnesses, like cardiovascular sickness, type 2 diabetes and malignant growths, are likewise hazard factors for some neurodegenerative infections. These danger factors incorporate a fatty eating regimen, nutrient inadequacies (for example folic corrosive and cell reinforcements) and an inactive way of life. Examination endeavors on neurodegenerative problems have quickly extended in the previous decade and those endeavors have prompted many promising restorative intercessions to increment both wellbeing length and life expectancy. Numerous individuals live for at least eighty years and appreciate a well-working cerebrum for the duration of their life expectancy. We subsequently realize that the human mind is fit for maturing effectively. We are currently at a phase where our insight into both the hereditary and ecological elements which have been connected to fruitless cerebrum maturing, and their phone and sub-atomic results, can be used to furnish everyone with guidance on maturing effectively. In this audit, we will examine two dietary systems, caloric limitation and intermittent fasting, which might actually be utilized to intervene fruitful maturing and prevent the beginning of certain neurodegenerative issues.

Dietary limitation and the sound maturing of man. Accepting Da Vinci's Man as a paragon of mankind we have depicted how he may live past the years ordinarily attributed to renaissance Homo sapiens through modifications in caloric admission. Both gross and cell physiology is significantly influenced by caloric limitation (CR) or intermittent fasting (IF) systems. As for net physiology there is obviously a critical decrease of muscle versus fat and mass, which upholds a solid cardiovascular framework and diminishes episodes of myocardial localized necrosis. Notwithstanding cardio security a more noteworthy resilience to stretch is incited in the liver, the supplement center of Homo sapiens. The presence of elective energy stores, for example, ketone bodies (for example beta-hydroxybutyrate) empower Homo sapiens to endure extra anxieties of life. Exorbitant and pernicious blood glucose is shortened by an upgraded affectability to insulin and glucose and its usage as a fuel source. The rise of neurotropic factors likewise upholds the support of complex neuronal circuits needed for memory maintenance and discernment. At the atomic level large numbers of the valuable impacts of CR/IF are restated. Proteins and nucleic acids are shielded from harming post-translational adjustments by means of up guidelines of sirtuin histone deacetylases and heat stun proteins (Hsp). To keep up Man during the useful times of fasting, peroxisome proliferator-actuated receptors (PPAR) are enacted to prepare fat stores for energy utilization. During these seasons of energy shortage, cell endurance is upheld by the enactment of fork head box-other (FoxO) record factors and through the age of neurotropic specialists, for example, mind determined neurotropic factor (BDNF). Incendiary cytokines, up controlled by CR/IF can even serve to permit improved synaptic strength during the hours of energy shortage.

1.2 Actions of Molecules Involved in Aging and Degeneration

An expanding number of hereditary and ecological variables are being distinguished that can deliver neurons helpless against the maturing cycle. A comprehension of how such causal or inclining hazard factors advance neuronal brokenness as well as death is basic for creating ways to deal with save useful neuronal circuits. Likewise, to other organ frameworks, cells in the mind experience a combined weight of oxidative and metabolic pressure that might be a widespread element of the maturing cycle. Expanded oxidative pressure during cerebrum maturing can be found in every one of the significant classes of cell particles, including proteins, lipids and nucleic acids. Some oxidative changes of proteins that have been seen in neurons during maturing incorporate carbonyl development, covalent adjustments of cysteine, and lysine and histidine deposits by the lipid peroxidation item 4-hydroxynonenal, nitration of proteins on tyrosine buildups, and glycation. A typical oxidative change of DNA, seen during mind maturing is the arrangement of 8-hydroxydeoxyguanosine. Every one of these changes of proteins, lipids and nucleic acids are additionally exacerbated in various degenerative problems like Alzheimer's infection (AD) and Parkinson's sickness (PD). Advertisement can be brought about by changes in the qualities encoding the amyloid forerunner protein (APP) as well as presenilin-1 (PS-1) or - 2 (PS-2). Every one of these changes brings about an expanded creation of amyloid-beta peptide which itself can build the oxidative weight on neurons. Advertisement prompts a reformist disintegration of psychological capacity with a deficiency of memory. Neuronal injury is consequently present in locales of the cerebrum that include the hippocampus and the cortex. Advertisement is portrayed by two principle obsessive trademarks that comprise of extracellular plaques of amyloid-beta peptide totals, and intracellular neurofibrillary tangles made out of the hyperphosphorylated microtubule-related protein tau. The beta-amyloid statement that comprises the plaques is made out of a 39–42 amino corrosive peptide, which is the proteolytic result of the APP protein. Curiously, the APP and presenilin changes have likewise been appeared to diminish levels of a discharged type of APP that has been appeared to advance synaptic pliancy (learning and memory) and endurance of neurons. PD is likewise a moderately regular reformist neurodegenerative issue influencing around 1% of the populace more seasoned than the age of 65 years and roughly 4–5% of the populace more established than the age of 85. It is brought about by a particular degeneration of the dopamine neurons in the substantia nigra. PD is portrayed by quake, unbending nature and gradualness of developments. Non-engine highlights, like dementia and dysautonomia, happen regularly, particularly in the high level phases of the sickness.

1.3 Health-Span and Life-Span Extension by Intermittent Fasting

Since forever, various social orders have perceived the advantageous consequences for wellbeing and general prosperity of restricting food consumption for specific timeframes, either for strict reasons or when food was scant. The principal generally perceived logical investigation of limited eating regimens and their capacity to expand life-range was distributed. It showed that taking care of subjects with an eating regimen containing inedible cellulose drastically broadened both mean and most extreme life expectancy in these creatures. Numerous investigations have affirmed this outcome and stretched out it to subject and different species including organic product flies nematodes, water bugs, arachnids and fish.

In this audit we will endeavor to demonstrate how, with dietary change, not exclusively life-length can be broadened yet in addition conceivably, wellbeing range, for example a great time wherein we have an illness/pathology free mien. We will likewise research through which sub-atomic components the advantages, in general living being, of dietary admission alteration are inferred. Varieties of this essential dietary system, presently known as caloric limitation (CR), are the best method of expanding the life expectancy of warm blooded animals without hereditarily adjusting them. All the more as of late, another variety of CR, intermittent fasting (IF) or each and every other day taking care of (EODF), has additionally been appeared to expand life-length and have advantageous wellbeing impacts. Subjects kept up on calorie-confined eating regimens are for the most part more modest and more slender and have less muscle versus fat and more modest significant organs than not indispensable took care of creatures. They are by and large more dynamic, which may identify with the need to look for food, and the typical age-related abatement in actual work is extraordinarily decreased in calorie-limited creatures. In any case, these creatures are more helpless against cold temperatures, which is a significant wellspring of mortality for little warm blooded animals (Berry and Bronson, 1992). The sum by which life-length is stretched out has been appeared to increment continuously as caloric admission is diminished, until the place of starvation. The hour of beginning of the dietary limitation (for example pre-or post-pubertal) and the term of the CR system additionally decide the sum by which life-range is broadened. Vitally both CR and IF can decrease the seriousness of hazard factors for sicknesses like diabetes and cardiovascular infection in subjects. In numerous examinations, execution of the IF dietary system brings about an around 20–30% decrease in caloric admission over the long haul. Upkeep of rats on this other day CR taking care of routine for 2–4 months brings about obstruction of hippocampal neurons to synthetically induced. In a water maze spatial learning task, this decreased damage to hippocampal neurons is also linked to a striking preservation of learning and memory. As a result, these dietary regimens may be beneficial for crippling and common neurodegenerative disorders like Alzheimer's, Huntington's, and Parkinson's disease.

1.4 Neuroprotection Molecular Mechanisms by Intermittent Fasting

Information from the creature considers depicted in this audit show that neurons in the cerebrums of subjects and subject kept up on CR or IF regimens display expanded protection from oxidative, metabolic and excitotoxic affronts. The basic inquiry to pose regarding these examinations is, what are the hidden atomic components that represent the insurance against this heap of intense cell affronts? Examiners have tended to this significant inquiry by estimating various proteins and lipids that are known to assume a part in ensuring neurons against a wide range of affronts. We will examine and exhibit what a complex physiological reaction to CR/IF happens in the living being and how this may in the long run mean sound maturing.

Responses of Stress

From nature we realize that the securing of accessible food structures quite possibly the most significant conduct sets and subsequently evacuation of sufficient food sources goes about as an extraordinary main thrust for engrained conduct and causes a specific level of mental and physiological pressure in the organic entity. This worldview, as with such countless parts of science, stretches out even to the basic physiological and cell measures inside the creature. To epitomize this, few distinctive pressure proteins have been estimated in the minds from subjects kept up on either not obligatory or CR eats less for a very long time. Instances of such pressure proteins incorporate warmth stun proteins and glucose-managed proteins. These atomic chaperone proteins associate with a wide range of proteins in cells and capacity to guarantee their legitimate collapsing, from one perspective, and corruption of harmed proteins, then again. They may likewise interface with, and adjust the capacity of, apoptotic proteins including caspases. Levels of a portion of these chaperone proteins might be expanded during the maturing interaction as a defensive reaction. Cell culture and in vivo examines have shown that heat-stun protein-70 (HSP-70) and glucose-controlled protein 78 (GRP-78) can secure neurons against injury and demise in trial models of neurodegenerative issues. Levels of HSP-70 and GRP-78 were discovered to be expanded in the cortical, hippocampal and striatal neurons of the CR subjects contrasted with the age-coordinated with not indispensable took care of creatures. Past examinations in this and different research centers have given proof that HSP-70 and GRP-78 can ensure neurons against excitotoxic and oxidative injury, which recommends that they add to the neuroprotective impact of CR. This information may exhibit that CR can prompt a gentle pressure reaction in neurons, probably because of a diminished energy, fundamentally glucose, accessibility. Notwithstanding these subcellular stress reactions, it has been accounted for that IF brings about expanded degrees of coursing corticosterone, which is typically related decidedly with the pressure condition of the creature. As opposed to impeding stressors, like constant wild pressure, which jeopardize neurons through glucocorticoid receptor actuation, intermittent fasting IF down directs glucocorticoid receptors with upkeep of mineralocorticoid receptors in neurons which can act to forestall neuronal harm and passing. It is possible that exchanging times of anabolism and catabolism, happening during IF, may assume an unthinking part in setting off expansions in cell stress obstruction and the maintenance of harmed proteins and cells.

Inordinate neurological pressure regularly appears as raised degrees of glutamatergic neurotransmission, for example in post ischemic occasions or epileptic seizures there can be an over-burden of cells with calcium, incited by the plain glutamate discharge that outcomes in possible cell passing. This type of excitoxic cell passing can be mirrored by the infusion of kainic corrosive (KA) into the cerebral ventricles/cerebrum areas of exploratory creatures. When the excitotoxic KA is infused into the dorsal hippocampus of subject it instigates seizures and harm to pyramidal neurons in areas CA3 and CA1. A critical expansion in the endurance of CA3 and CA1 neurons in the IF subject contrasted and subject took care of not indispensable, after the kainic affront has been illustrated.

Neurotropic Factors

As both IF and CR prompt a gentle pressure reaction in synapses this can bring about the initiation of repaying instruments, for example the up guideline of neurotropic factors, for example, BDNF and glial cell line-inferred neurotropic factor (GDNF) just as the previously mentioned heat stun proteins. On the off chance that regimens have been shown to enhance and lessen neuronal harm and improve the useful result in creature models of neurological injury, for example, stroke and furthermore neurodegenerative issues like Parkinson's infection, and Huntington's illness. The neuroprotective component of IF isn't known, yet it has been accounted for that IF prompts the creation of cerebrum determined neurotropic factor (BDNF) which was related with expanded hippocampal neurogenesis in subjects and subject. One of the essential neuroprotective systems ascribed to BDNF gives off an impression of being the capacity of BDNF-intervened enactment of its related TrkB receptor which at that point entrains incitement of numerous flagging pathways. Noticeable among these TrkB flagging pathways is the phosphatidyl inositol 3-kinase (PI3K)/protein kinase B (Akt) pathway that has been embroiled in a few of the CR/IF defensive components that will be examined at more noteworthy length in this audit.

Ketone bodies

Dietary fasting is known to bring about an expanded creation of ketone bodies, for example beta-hydroxybutyrate, which can be utilized by the creature as a fuel source notwithstanding restricted glucose accessibility. Regarding ketogenesis apparently IF regimens appear to be more agreeable to this energy creation pathway than more exacting CR conventions. Subject on IF regimens have been appeared to burden normal more than subject on CR regimens. They likewise have bigger fat stores and a more prominent ketogenic reaction than CR subject. On the off chance that dietary systems can build up a two-overlay expansion in the fasting serum centralization of beta-hydroxybutyrate contrasted and subject took care of not indispensable. This shift to ketogenesis may assume an immediate part in the cytoprotective impacts of IF, in light of the fact that it has been accounted for that subjects took care of a ketogenic diet show expanded protection from seizures, and that beta-hydroxybutyrate itself can ensure neurons in subjects of Alzheimer's and Parkinson's infections. Ketogenic counts calories, which advance a metabolic shift from glucose usage to ketogenesis, are additionally recommended for certain patients with epilepsy as this is prophylactic against the reformist excitotoxic neuronal harm and debasement that can happen if the condition is untreated.

Glucose and Insulin Signaling

During fasting or dietary limitation the essential adjustment to the creature is the accessibility of glucose for oxidative breath. The systems by which energy is gotten from substitute sources or how the leftover glucose is taken care of are fitting to the extrapolation of the medical advantages of CR/IF regimens. The significance of glucose taking care of proficiency for sound maturing can be exhibited by the way that glucose levels in the blood, incorporated over the long haul, have been proposed to prompt undeniable degrees of non-enzymatic glycation, a type of protein harm. CR has been appeared to explicitly constrict oxyradical creation and harm and non-enzymatic glycation.

Both IF and CR regimens effectsly affect insulin and glucose levels, for example decrease, yet curiously they effectsly affect serum IGF-1 levels and serum beta-hydroxybutyrate levels, for example both these boundaries are expanded with intermittent fasting IF contrasted with CR. A longitudinal report on male subjects exhibited that CR diminished the mean 24-h plasma glucose focus by around 15 mg/dl and the insulin fixation by about half. CR system creatures used glucose at similar rate as did the subjects took care of not indispensable, notwithstanding the lower plasma glucose and especially lower plasma insulin levels. Hence, it is suggested that CR either expands glucose adequacy or insulin responsiveness or both, and that the support of low degrees of glucose and insulin control the useful and life-broadening activities of CR. CR has likewise been found to lessen plasma glucose and insulin fixations in fasting rhesus monkeys. Furthermore, CR can build insulin affectability in rhesus and cynomolgus monkeys. A significant justification this accentuation being set on the insulin–glucose control framework in maturing is the finding that deficiency of-work changes of the insulin flagging framework bring about existence augmentation in three species: C. elegans, D. melanogaster, and subject. Generally, from numerous test studies, CR and IF appear to persistently lessen the flowing degrees of insulin bringing about an inevitable improved glucose preparation and an upgraded insulin affectability, the two of which serve to keep a stockpile of glucose for the essential organs, focal sensory system and balls to help these basic organs on schedule of restricted energy admission. The genuine decrease of insulin receptor flagging interceded by diminished plasma insulin levels has an effect additionally on a few different elements that significantly sway upon the cell reaction to CR/IF; this will be examined in later segments.

Cytokines

There is mounting proof to recommend that provocative cycles could be fundamentally associated with the improvement old enough related pathologies, for example, those saw in Alzheimer's sickness. The enactment of microglia in light of injury or during maturing causes the acceptance of a fiery like reaction. This reaction is exemplified and started by an improved articulation of interleukin-1 in the animated microglia. Considering this it is hence obvious that fiery cytokines may likewise be ensnared in the CR/IF-interceded measures that improve this neurodegeneration. Late discoveries recommend that IFN is a significant go between of neuronal pliancy, for example IFN may improve synaptogenesis, direct synaptic pliancy and control neurogenesis.

It was as of late revealed that degrees of IFN are expanded in flowing leukocytes of monkeys that had been kept up on a CR diet. It has additionally been shown that CR lifts the statement of IFN in the hippocampus where it applies an excitoprotective activity of IFN. Cytokines can likewise be delivered by instinctive organs outside the insusceptible framework and the focal sensory system. Fat tissue, which amasses during maturing and is explicitly diminished upon CR or IF regimens, can go about as an endocrine organ, which produces trophic chemicals that are dynamic all through the body, for example tumor putrefaction factor (TNF). TNF has additionally been appeared to trigger insulin opposition in creatures. In vitro cell-culture examines have shown that TNF renders cells insulin safe through a down guideline of glucose carrier union just as through obstruction with insulin receptor flagging pathways which we have seen are fundamentally engaged with sound maturing. In vivo, the shortfall of the TNF receptor essentially improves insulin affectability which copies the insulin-related impacts found in CR/IF creatures. Curiously, it has been shown that CR constricts the age-related up guideline of atomic factor (NF), which is a record factor that initiates the statement of TNF in fat tissue and the creation of fiery cytokines in resistant cells. In this way constriction of TNF instigated insulin obstruction may upgrade the glucose use limit of the organic entity, subsequently fighting off the unfavorable impacts of exorbitant blood glucose that may happen in the midst of chronic weakness and with propelling age.

Adipose and Satiety-Generated hormones

Leptin and adiponectin are two chemicals that are normally connected with the input control of hunger and satiety. Both of these variables are created by fat tissue which is obviously significantly influenced by CR/IF systems. Notwithstanding its job in satiety, leptin, delivered into the dissemination, diminishes the degree of stress chemicals and builds thyroid action and thyroid-chemical levels which both outcome in expanded energy use. As we have seen, CR regimens will in general up manage pressure chemicals in an okay way and moreover they can down control thyroid chemicals, possibly through this constriction of flowing leptin levels. Anyway leptin's part in interceding the valuable impacts of CR might be optional to its satiety job as it has been shown that subject that need leptin lamentably exhibit a decreased life expectancy, contrasted with not obligatory creatures, and are corpulent. Adiponectin has been appeared to trigger expanded insulin affectability by means of up guideline of AMP-initiated protein kinase. This kinase directs glucose and fat digestion in muscle in light of energy limit, and has been appeared to secure neurons against metabolic pressure. Significantly, adiponectin levels ascend during CR, which recommends that this fat determined chemical may likewise have a significant contributory job in the physiological shift to an upgraded insulin affectability in these creatures. Late discoveries show that subject that have been hereditarily designed to be lean live more. Surely, tissue-explicit knockout of the insulin receptor in fat cells keeps the tissue from putting away fat, which brings about lean creatures that live altogether more than wild-type subject. These information propose that instinctive fat may be particularly significant in driving insulin obstruction and pathogenesis.

Sirtuins

As lower life forms, for example yeast and nematode worms, have an impressively more limited life expectancy than well evolved creatures they have demonstrated valuable for the revelation of the atomic determinants of sound life span. It has gotten evident that among the different variables that have been recognized that control life-range in these lower organic entities, a considerable lot of these additionally interface the change of caloric admission to the expansion in wellbeing length so wanted by dietary mediations of sickness measures.

One of the essential hereditary determinants of replicative life expectancy to rise out of hereditary examinations in yeast is the quiet data controller 2 (SIR2). The SIR2 quality was meant on the grounds that it intercedes a particular quality hushing activity. Inhibitory changes of SIR2 can abbreviate life-range, and expanded quality measurements of SIR2 broadened life-length. The SIR2 ortholog in C. elegans was correspondingly demonstrated to be a vital determinant of the life expectancy around there. As yeast and C. elegans separated from a typical precursor around one billion years prior this may propose that relatives of that predecessor, including warm blooded animals, will have SIR2-related qualities engaged with controlling their life expectancy. As dietary guideline has additionally demonstrated to be an amazing modulator of life expectancy it is sensible to guess that CR/IF and SIR2 qualities may join to assume a significant part in these numerous and complex physiological pathways. Mammalian homologues of the yeast SIR2 quality have in this way been found and strangely the SIR2 ortholog, SIRT1, may to a limited extent intervene an expansive cluster of physiological impacts that happen in creatures on a changed eating routine, beit CR or IF. The group of proteins found that are encoded for by the mammalian SIR2 homologues are all in all named sirtuins. A few late reports have shown increments in SIRT1 protein levels because of food hardship. Furthermore SIR up guideline has been appeared in light of cell stressors, like high osmolarity, subsequently the sirtuin group of proteins could be effectively directed by the gentle, controllable pressure initiated by CR/IF. Sirtuins have a moderately uncommon enzymatic limit as they are NAD-subordinate histone deacetylases. The mammalian SIRT1 quality item chemical can, notwithstanding histones, deacetylate numerous different substrates. In such manner, SIRT1 was as of late appeared to deacetylate and down regulate NF. It is interesting to guess that the up guideline of SIRT1 by CR adds to the noticed expansion in insulin affectability and decrease in irritation, conceivably through the control of the NF/TNF pathways.

It have proposed an atomic pathway for SIR2 enactment that possibly interfaces modifications in caloric admission to life-range expansion. Upon CR/IF there is an underlying expansion in oxygen utilization and breath, to the detriment of fermentative cycles. Maturation is a commonplace component by which cells can create ATP and furthermore store overabundance energy as ethanol when glucose is plentiful. This metabolic shift triggers an attending decrease in NADH levels. NADH goes about as a serious inhibitor of SIR2, so its decrease during CR/IF periods would be required to up manage the compound and subsequently broaden the organic entity's life expectancy in accordance with yeast and C. elegans considers. Steady with this, removal of mitochondrial electron transport hindered the impact of CR on life-range, and overexpressing NADH dehydrogenase, the compound that shunts electrons from NADH to the electron transport chain, expanded the creature's life expectancy. Hence it shows up then that CR/IF initiates a more effective utilization of glucose by means of an increment in breath. Notwithstanding this there is a change in muscle cells from utilizing glucose, which is somewhat, processed in not indispensable creatures fermentatively (delivering lactate), at the utilization of unsaturated fats, which are oxidatively used. This shift saves glucose for the mind, forestalling neurodegeneration, and connects with the trademark upgrade of insulin affectability in muscle and liver found in CR. Albeit the activities of sirtuins in the sensory system are simply starting to be investigated, it has been accounted for that SIR2 (SIRT1 in vertebrates) actuation through expanded quality measurements or treatment with the sirtuin activator resveratrol can secure neurons against the pathogenic impacts of polyglutamine-extended huntingtin proteins in worm and mouse models of Huntington's infection.

Sirtuins likewise appear to assume a part in interceding the successful job of fat tissue in the physiological transaction of the advantages of CR/IF systems to the living being. Perhaps the main controllers of fat tissue work is the peroxisome proliferator-actuated record factor receptor gamma. This receptor goes about as an atomic record factor that controls numerous qualities associated with cell endurance and reactions to metabolic changes. One PPAR quality objective, the aP2 quality, encodes a protein that helps fat stockpiling. SIRT1 can go about as a repressor of PPAR, in this way down directing qualities, for example, the mouse aP2 quality. During fasting SIRT1 enactment is trailed by an improved restricting to the aP2 advertiser in fat tissue. This causes a restraint of aP2 quality articulation causing a possible advancement of fat assembly into the blood to help the life form's energy balance. Endless supply of caloric admission there is a traditionalist enactment of SIRT1 in fat tissue, which acts to lessen fat stores and likely resets hormonal levels to change the speed of maturing. This methodology likewise bodes well when it is viewed as that effective proliferation is additionally managed by muscle versus fat and is stopped during CR, possibly to continue when accessible energy supplies become more bountiful.

Peroxisome proliferator-activated receptor and co-factors

PPARs, as we have seen, are individuals from the atomic chemical receptor subfamily of record factors. PPARs structure useful heterodimers with retinoid X receptors (RXRs) and these heterodimers manage record of different qualities. There are three known subtypes of PPARs. These atomic receptor record factors manage qualities associated with supplement transport and digestion just as protection from stress. PPARs themselves additionally enlist different proteins notwithstanding the RXR to intercede their total capacity. One such protein is the peroxisome proliferator-actuated receptor (PPAR) co-activator 1 (PGC-1). This co-activator has been demonstrated to be firmly managed by dietary change in lower creatures and higher warm blooded animals.

PGC-1 exists in two isoforms, and these isoforms have arisen as unmistakable controllers of the versatile reactions to caloric hardship. PGC-1 manages the ligand-subordinate and - free initiation of an enormous number of atomic receptors including the PPARs. There has been accounted for an age-subordinate decrease in PGC-1 which may fuel the maturing cycle. Anyway in subject and primates CR has been appeared to invert this age-subordinate decline in PGC-1, PPAR and directed qualities

PGC-1, the main PGC relative recognized was described as a protein that associates with the PPAR to manage earthy colored fat separation during variation to cold pressure. This virus stress might be viewed as closely resembling the physiological and mental pressure instigated by caloric limitation. During CR/IF periods, when insulin levels are low, PGC-1 and PGC-1 beta quality articulation is improved in subjects. PGC-1 was likewise prompted in the livers of subject and subjects after longer term CR. PGC-1 and beta can coordinately direct qualities associated with gluconeogenesis and unsaturated fat beta-oxidation in various organs during fasting. Both these cycles are useful to the upkeep of a sound energy balance in the midst of restricted food. Thus through PPAR initiation additional provisions of glucose can be assembled and substitute fuel sources can be misused. Just as PGC guideline during fasting, PPAR is additionally up directed by fasting in liver, little and digestive organ, thymus and pancreas. Countless qualities engaged with unsaturated fat beta-oxidation, known to be directed by PPAR are likewise expanded in articulation because of fasting. During times of fasting PPAR take out subject show a powerlessness to direct qualities associated with unsaturated fat beta-and oxidation and ketogenesis in the liver, kidney and heart alongside absence of control of blood levels of glucose or ketone bodies.

Not exclusively is the liver the energy-directing center of warm blooded animals however it additionally addresses perhaps the main stores of glycogen, supplements and nutrients. One would accordingly anticipate that there would be a basic connection between adjustments of caloric admission and resultant hepatic capacity. Along these lines it has been shown that CR shields the liver from a wide scope of natural stressors, a significant number of which instigate harm through flowing fiery arbiters. PPAR has been appeared to direct hepatic reactions to different types of pressure. Subject pre-presented to PPAR agonists show diminished cell harm, expanded tissue fix, and diminished mortality after openness to various physical and synthetic hepatic stressors. Apparently utilitarian PPAR are vital for the CR-intervened assurance of the liver from harm instigated by hepatotoxicants like thioacetamide. In particular, it was shown by that PPAR take out subject, as opposed to wild-type subject, were not shielded from thioacetamide by CR systems. Lipid peroxide levels, related with oxidative cell stress in the fringe and the focal sensory system, are likewise altogether expanded in maturing. PPAR take out subject show a checked height in lipid peroxidation items contrasted with wild-type subject. Hence PPAR may impact maturing through the guideline of various harm and fix measures after openness to a plenty of endogenous or natural stressors.

PGC-1 isoforms are transcriptionally or post transnationally directed in well evolved creatures by a few flagging pathways embroiled in the association between CR/IF and life-length augmentation. These incorporate fork head box "other" (FoxO) record factors (through an insulin/insulin-like development factor-I - subordinate pathway), glucagon-invigorated cell AMP (cAMP) reaction component restricting protein (CREB), stress-enacted protein kinases (p38 and N-terminal kinase) and obviously SIRT1. We will talk about next how these elements connect to control the atomic instruments of CR/IF that sway upon interpretation to sound maturing.

Transcription Factors of FoxO

In warm blooded animals, insulin and IGF-I tie to one or the other insulin or IGF-1 receptors initiating different flagging pathways. Regarding the maturing interaction and the improvement of degenerative issues it appears to be that the main pathway entrained by insulin/IGF-1 is the standard phosphatidylinositol 3-kinase and serine–threonine protein kinases (Akt-1/Akt-2/protein kinase B [PKB]) flagging course. In C. elegans, this pathway decides reactions to life span and natural pressure. Transformations in C. elegans which inactivate the insulin/IGF-I pathway, including Daf-2, the receptor for insulin/IGF-I or the PI3K ortholog Age-1, increment life-range just as temperature and oxidative anxieties. These impacts require inversion of negative guideline of the pressure obstruction factor, Daf-16. Daf-16 encodes a record factor containing a "forkhead" DNA restricting space. Overexpression of Daf-16 in worms or an ortholog in flies essentially broadens their life expectancy. Daf-16 directs the declaration of a variety of qualities engaged with xenobiotic digestion and stress obstruction. Mammalian homologs of Daf-16 fall into the group of FoxO factors. There are four primary gatherings of mammalian FoxOs, FoxO1, FoxO3, FoxO4 and FoxO6. FoxO record factors have a place with the bigger Forkhead group of proteins, a group of transcriptional controllers portrayed by the preserved 'forkhead box' DNA-restricting area. These FoxO proteins control a wide cluster of qualities that all are connected by a typical component in that they serve to control energy metabolim in the organic entity because of ecological changes, for example limitation of accessible food. For instance FoxOs control qualities engaged with glucose digestion (glucose 6-phosphatase); cell passing (Fas-ligand), responsive oxygen species detoxification (catalse and manganese superoxide dismutase) and DNA fix (development capture and DNA harm inducible protein 45 and harm explicit DNA-restricting protein 1).

Insulin receptor incitement, during caloric admission, prompts enactment of the PI3K/Akt pathway and resultant phosphorylation of FoxOs in warm blooded animals. Phosphorylated FoxO factors are perceived by 14-3-3 proteins which work with their vehicle out of the core, decreasing their transcriptional action. Subsequently upon CR/IF there is an unpredictable transaction among enactment and inactivation of these FoxO factors. There are conceivably useful impacts of FoxO enactment and inactivation relying on the predominant cell conditions. Mammalian FoxO relatives complete capacities that decide cell endurance during seasons of pressure including guideline of apoptosis, cell-cycle designated spot control, and oxidative pressure opposition. Initiation of FoxO3 or FoxO4 prompts expansions in cell-cycle G1 capture and expansions in apoptosis probably as an approach to dispense with cells harmed by oxidative pressure. Hence changes in the ability to initiate the PI3K/Akt pathways can have emotional impacts upon cell survivability and this cycle might be basic in moving the beneficial outcomes of CR/IF to the living being. CR uncouples insulin/IGF-I motioning to FoxO factors by especially lessening plasma

IGF-I and insulin levels in subjects. These declines in coursing insulin/IGF-I levels result in diminished Akt phosphorylation in liver and diminished PI3K articulation in muscle. Moreover there is a compensatory expansion in the declaration of FoxO relatives by fasting or CR. Accordingly, when insulin flagging is diminished, for example during CR/IF there are expansions in atomic/cytoplasmic FoxO proportions however FoxO factor articulation also. By and large, numerous examinations have uncovered that down guideline of insulin/IGF-I flagging outcomes in expansions in the action of FoxO factors, that fundamentally direct cell endurance instruments, and that these changes are discovered reliably in numerous assorted models of life span among various species.

A significant number of the qualities directed by FoxOs are comparatively controlled by the tumor silencer p53, which has prompted the theory that these two qualities may work in show to forestall both injurious maturing and tumor development. Steady with this chance, p53 and FoxO are both phosphorylated and acetylated because of oxidative pressure boosts and UV radiations. Moreover, both p53 and FoxOs tie to SIRT1 deacetylase. FoxO and p53 appear to be practically connected as p53 can restrain FoxO work by actuating serum and glucocorticoid instigated kinase (SGK) - interceded phosphorylation of FoxO3 bringing about its movement from the core to the cytoplasm. FoxO3 has been found to forestall p53 from subduing SIRT1 quality articulation. FoxO-instigated suppression of p53 has all the earmarks of being interceded by the immediate cooperation somewhere in the range of FoxO3 and p53. That FoxO factors instigate SIRT1 articulation is steady with the perception that SIRT1 articulation is expanded in rat tissues when insulin and IGF-1 are brought down by CR. Thusly, SIRT1 itself can tie to and deacetylate p53 and FoxO record factors, controlling their movement. Subject holding a change, which brings about the actuation of p53, show a critical decrease of life expectancy and display indications of untimely maturing. Curiously, while initiation of p53 in these mouse models lessens life-range, p53 actuation actually permits an expanded protection from malignancy, exhibiting that p53 cause tumor concealment to the detriment of life span.

Perhaps the main ongoing fields of caloric limitation study is the exhibition that CR might have the option to forestall the age of various types of disease itself. For instance, in subject with hereditarily lessened p53 levels CR expanded the idleness of unconstrained tumor improvement (for the most part lymphomas) by around 75%. It is hence certain that there is an unobtrusive and confounded connection between these connected variables that are connected together by changes in dietary energy consumption.

Notwithstanding adverse guideline by insulin/IGF-1 flagging and p53, FoxO factors are managed by the CREB restricting protein (CBP) and a connected protein, p300. Curiously, cell overexpression of CBP or p300 improves the capacity of FoxO variables to actuate useful quality articulation. SIRT1 again appears to assume a focal part in versatile changes to energy guideline as it can turn around the negative guideline of FoxO relatives by CBP. Like PGC-1, SIRT1 levels are expanded during CR in subject liver and are contrarily directed by insulin and IGF-I. Moreover, the connected relative SIRT3, a mitochondrial protein, shows expanded articulation in white and earthy colored fat upon CR.

FoxOs appear to exist at a nexus between instruments that associate cell stress reactions to possible endurance components. For example the pressure related protein kinase cJun N-terminal kinase 1 (JNK-1), which fills in as an atomic sensor for different stressors effectively can handle FoxO transcriptional activity. In C. elegans, JNK-1 straightforwardly cooperates with and phosphorylates the FoxO homologue Daf-16, and because of warmth stress, JNK-1 advances the movement of Daf-16 into the core. Overexpression of JNK-1 in C. elegans prompts expansions in life-range and expanded endurance after heat pressure. In D. melanogaster also, gentle actuation of JNK prompts expanded pressure resilience and life span reliant upon a flawless FoxO.

Taking everything into account it appears to be that FoxO record factors are promising contender to fill in as sub-atomic connections between dietary adjustments and life span. In conditions like CR/IF where the flowing degrees of insulin/IGF-1 are constricted to improve euglycemia, FoxO atomic movement brings about the upregulation of a progression of target qualities that advance cell cycle capture, stress obstruction, and apoptosis. Outer distressing improvements additionally trigger the relocalization of FoxO factors into the core, subsequently permitting a versatile reaction to push upgrades. Steady with the idea that pressure opposition is profoundly combined with life-length expansion, actuation of FoxO record factors in worms and flies builds life span. FoxO proteins decipher natural upgrades, including the pressure initiated by caloric limitation into changes in quality articulation programs that may arrange organismal sound maturing and possible life span.

1.5 Intermittent Fasting and Caloric restriction in Humans

We are moving toward a complete comprehension of the different sub-atomic systems by which changes in caloric admission can be moved to an improved endurance of cells during the maturing cycle. Anyway the inquiry remains whether CR and IF will affect people. Until this point in time, there have been no all-around controlled logical examinations to decide the impacts of long haul CR on people. As of now there are considers progressing including 30% CR in non-human primates (rhesus monkeys) and information so distant from these investigations look encouraging, in that they have upheld the life-and wellbeing expanding properties of this dietary system.

In any case, the inordinate loss of muscle versus fat and the accompanying decrease in sex steroids can prompt feminine inconsistencies, amenorrhea, bone diminishing and the improvement of osteoporosis in females. Maybe a variety of the CR/IF conventions in which there is a milder caloric limitation joined with an adjustment of taking care of recurrence may have a more prominent probability of consistence among human subjects. Ideally this more delicate adjustment of dietary food admission will in any case hold the advantages of the trial systems utilized up until now. It is important that to date most examinations utilizing CR have contrasted the gainful impacts of CR with overweight (or even fat) age-coordinated with control creatures. It is muddled whether creatures with a sound bodyweight, that can participate in normal exercise and have some type of mental incitement (as they would do in the wild), would profit by a CR system. Ongoing investigations did with human subjects, subject to 25% CR, are anyway endeavoring to address this as they are utilizing control subjects with ordinary weight records.

The advancement of a substance CR mimetic might be a promising helpful road for the treatment of neurodegenerative illnesses and to defer the maturing cycle, as it would give comparative medical advantages to CR, (for example, expanding wellbeing and life expectancy), while going around the drawn out need to lessen food consumption. Notwithstanding, it stays not yet clear whether a CR mimetic would be a doable medication to deliver, particularly since the enthusiasm for the cycles whereby CR applies its defensive impacts are still fairly deficient and the fundamental components are ending up being perplexing. One should likewise not markdown the mental impacts of food admission in higher, more contemplative, creatures like people. We have a practically special enthusiastic association with an enormous assortment of staples. Consequently expulsion of this mental help, during a CR/IF-like system may mostly balance the physiological advantages of these ideal models.

The principle factor that may invalidate the far reaching execution of CR/IF as a compelling geronto-remedial is possibly the advanced Western way of life of close to steady work and industriously high feelings of anxiety. Henceforth, to fabricate the general public and innovative advances that we are utilized to, we have left behind the taking care of examples of our old progenitors for steady mental movement and restricted actual exercise. Because of expansions in our everyday movement we have an expanded energy (predominantly glucose) necessity while our physiology is generally still equipped to a dining experience and starvation example of energy consumption normal for our agrarian Homo sapiens precursors. This difficulty between our advanced society/conduct and our antiquated physiology will address a common issue for gerontology for quite a long time to come. Ideally, with our quickly propelling enthusiasm for our maturing interaction we won't have to trust that our physiological advancement will find our way of life.

Chapter 2. Intermittent Fasting and Reduced Meal Frequency

In spite of the fact that utilization of 3 suppers/d is the most widely recognized example of eating in industrialized nations, a logical reasoning for this feast recurrence regarding ideal wellbeing is deficient. An eating routine with less supper recurrence can improve the wellbeing and expand the life expectancy of research facility creatures, yet its impact on people has never been tried. A pilot study was directed to build up the impacts of a decreased dinner recurrence diet on wellbeing markers in solid, typical weight grown-ups. The examination was a randomized hybrid plan with two multi week treatment periods. During the treatment time frames, subjects devoured the entirety of the calories required for weight upkeep in either 3 suppers/d or 1 feast/d.

2.1 Introduction

Gorging is a significant reason for dreariness and mortality in people, and, likewise, caloric limitation has different medical advantages for the large. Caloric limitation may likewise improve the strength of people who are not viewed as overweight. While supplement thick, low-calorie eats less carbs have various medical advantages, the impact of dinner recurrence on wellbeing has not been set up. In any case, investigations of different research center creatures and explicitly of subjects have shown that dietary limitation (caloric limitation or intermittent fasting long haul intermittent fasting on account of subjects) can expand life expectancy and secure against or stifle infection measures liable for cardiovascular sickness (CVD), disease, diabetes, and neurodegenerative issues. The last investigations showed valuable impacts of intermittent fasting on circulatory strain, glucose digestion, and weakness of cardiovascular and synapses to injury. Notwithstanding an overall insight among people in general everywhere that it is critical to eat 3 dinners/d, no controlled investigations have straightforwardly looked at the impacts of various feast frequencies on human wellbeing. This information hole has been recognized by the 2005 Dietary Guidelines Advisory Committee Report as a future exploration heading.

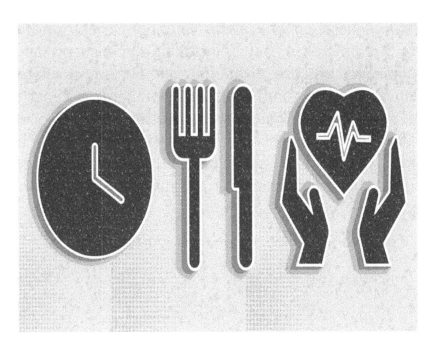

Investigations of subjects and monkeys have prompted a few theories concerning the cell and atomic systems whereby dietary limitation expands life expectancy and ensures against infection. The oxidative pressure speculation recommends that maturing and age-related sicknesses result from combined oxidative harm to proteins, lipids, and nucleic acids; by diminishing the measure of oxyradicals delivered in mitochondria, dietary limitation impedes maturing and illness. A subsequent theory is that dietary limitation is helpful principally due to its impacts on energy digestion; i.e., it expands insulin affectability. A third speculation, which may have a specific connection to the useful impacts of diminished dinner recurrence/intermittent fasting, is that dietary limitation actuates a gentle cell stress reaction in which cells up-manage the statement of qualities that empower them to adapt to serious pressure. A few physiologic factors have been appeared to change in

157

creatures kept up on caloric limitation or intermittent fasting regimens (or both), including diminished plasma insulin and glucose fixations, diminished circulatory strain and pulse, and improved invulnerable capacity. The current pilot study was directed to decide the attainability of controlled supper recurrence in ordinary weight, moderately aged people. A few physiologic results and biomarkers of wellbeing were likewise examined.

2.2 Methods and Subjects

Sound people matured 40–50 y were enlisted by paper ad from the more prominent Washington, DC, metropolitan region. Incorporation in the investigation depended on a weight record (BMI; in kg) somewhere in the range of 18 and 25 and a typical eating example of 3 dinners/d. Subjects were rejected on the off chance that they detailed tobacco use, late pregnancy or lactation, history of CVD or drug use for CVD, hypertension, diabetes, mental condition, malignancy, or work in high-hazard occupations (this last avoidance basis was because of the potential for wooziness or shortcoming during the dinner skipping stage). Study passage was endorsed by a doctor based on clinical history, blood and pee test screening results, and an actual assessment.

Study Design

This examination was a randomized hybrid plan with two multi week treatment periods. During the treatment time frames, subjects burned-through the entirety of their calories for weight support circulated in either 3 dinners/d (control diet) or 1 supper/d (test diet). A multi week waste of time period was incorporated between medicines. The control diet comprised of 3 suppers/d (breakfast, lunch, and supper) and the test "dinner skipping" (or 1 feast/d) diet comprised of a similar every day allocation of food eaten inside a 4 hours' time frame in the early evening. The subjects were taken care of at an energy consumption that would keep up body weight so feast recurrence would be the lone significant change in their eating routine over the span of the investigation. The examination was a communitarian exertion between the US Department of Agriculture, Beltsville Human Nutrition Research Center (BHNRC; Beltsville, MD), and the National Institute on Aging.

Study Diets

Every day, subjects burned-through supper at the BHNRC Human Study Facility under the oversight of an enlisted dietitian. Toward the finish of supper, subject dinner plate were examined to guarantee total utilization of the food. All morning meals and snacks were pressed for complete. Just food sources given by the Human Study Facility were permitted to be devoured during the examination. A 7 days menu pattern of ordinary American food varieties was detailed by utilizing nutritionist.

During the initial fourteen days of the investigation, subjects haphazardly appointed to the 1 supper/d eating routine were taken care of 2 dinners/d (lunch and supper); for the following a month and a half, all food was burned-through somewhere in the range of 1700 and 2100, which made a base quick of 20 h/d. While keeping up the equivalent macronutrient dissemination among test and control diets, breakfast and lunch food things were fill in for customary evening feast things. Energy-thick food varieties were picked to help with decreasing the volume of food to be burned-through.

Subjects were permitted limitless measures of sans calorie food varieties like water, espresso (without sugar or milk), diet sodas, salt, and pepper. A multi day crisis supply of food that met the examination convention was given to each expose to use during any severe climate. Subjects were needed to burn-through the entirety of the food sources and just the food varieties given by the

Human Study Facility at determined occasions during the controlled taking care of periods.

Body weight was estimated each day prior to the evening supper, when subjects showed up at the office. So that subjects could keep up consistent body weight during the investigation, energy admission was changed in 200-kcal increases. Energy prerequisites for weight upkeep were determined by utilizing the Harris-Benedict recipe, which gauges basal energy use, and duplicated by a movement factor of 1.3–1.5. This recipe has demonstrated effective in assessing weight-upkeep energy necessities at our office. Subjects finished an everyday poll in regards to their overall wellbeing; any utilization of remedy or over-the-counter prescriptions; factors identified with dietary consistence; and exercise played out; the survey likewise offered subjects the chance to write in inquiries of their own about the eating regimen. Subjects were urged to keep up their ordinary exercise routine all through the examination.

Physiologic Evaluations

Physiologic factors estimated were pulse, pulse, internal heat level, and body piece. These estimations were gathered at standard, a month, and toward the finish of every one of the 2 treatment time frames. Momentarily, subjects were situated in a tranquil space for 5 min, and circulatory strain and pulse were estimated multiple times with a Dinamap Compact Monitor. Internal heat level was estimated on either a Dinamap or a compact oral computerized thermometer. Body organization was estimated by utilizing bioelectrical impedance investigation (BIA). Subjects abstained and avoided substantial exercise before these estimations. Abstract satiety and appetite were evaluated day by day before utilization of the evening dinner, in both the trial and control slims down, by utilizing 4 visual simple scales (VASs) that depicted yearning, want to eat, the measure of food that could be eaten, and stomach completion. The VASs were every one of the 100-mm long, and they were moored at one or the flip side with terms demonstrating inverse descriptors.

Analysis of Biological Sample

Blood was gathered at benchmark, a month, and the finish of every one of the 2 treatment time frames after at least 12 h of fasting. The entirety of the standard examples were gathered in the first part of the day. The a month and end-of-treatment tests were gathered toward the beginning of the day from subjects following the control diet and in the evening (before supper) from subjects following the 1 feast/d eating regimen. Also, as a proportion of consistence, blood tests were gathered at unannounced occasions on 3 events from the subjects when they were burning-through 1 supper/d and were broke down for fasting blood glucose and triacylglycerol focuses. The gathered blood tests were utilized to plan 0.8–2.0-mL aliquots of plasma, serum, and red platelets that were put away at short 80 °C in cryovials. Test examinations incorporated a lipid profile, an extensive metabolic board, and total blood tally (CBC), and cortisol fixation. Investigations were performed at the Core Laboratory of the public foundations of wellbeing) and at clinical lab by utilizing standard strategies and quality-control measures from the clinical research facility improvement changes. Plasma absolute cholesterol, HDL cholesterol, and triacylglycerol were estimated enzymatically with business units on 250 analyzer. LDL-cholesterol focuses were determined by utilizing the condition. Serum cortisol focuses were investigated on an immunoassay analyzer (with CVs of 5.3% and 7.2%, individually).

Assessment of Physical Activity

Actual work observing (PAM) was surveyed with the utilization of the Actigraph accelerometer throughout 7 days to acquire the normal day by day and week by week action checks. Estimations were acquired during week 2 (benchmark) and week 7 (finish of treatment) of every treatment period. Subjects were told to wear the movement screen as long as conceivable consistently. The movement screen, worn as a cozily fitting belt around the midriff with the producer's "score" confronting vertically, was set to peruse the information in 1-min portions. Subjects were approached to wear the screen on the correct hip, except if they revealed being not able to do as such. Notwithstanding the action screen position, each subject wore the screen on a similar side and at a similar area all through the examination. As well as wearing the screens, subjects kept a little day by day log to detail the occasions when the screen was worn, the exercises that were done when the screen was not worn (i.e., dozing or showering), and any activity performed (if the screen was worn). In every one of the treatment time frames, subjects were approached to wear the screen for 9 days, fully intent on getting 7 entire long periods of information. In the event that a subject detailed not wearing the action screen for a given day, the person in question was approached to wear the screen an additional day.

Active work information got from the Actigraph accelerometer were handled by utilizing a strategy created in our office. Momentarily, most subjects commonly eliminate the screens occasionally during the day or around evening time for rest (or both). Investigations from our lab show that these missing information focuses can detrimentally affect the forecast of active work, so we built up a methodology that treats each checking day as a 24-hours day regardless of how long the screen was worn on quickly. Screen records are filtered by a program that assesses the time spent dozing and credits a consistent incentive for those occasions. Other missing strings of information 20 min long are "filled in" by attribution, based on the screen evacuation times announced in the log. These information preparing strategies significantly diminish the inconstancy intrinsic with movement screen information.

Analysis of Stats

An examination of change (ANOVA) fitting for a 2-period hybrid investigation with rehashed measures inside period was utilized to assess supper recurrence impacts on result factors utilizing the blended method in programming. The factual model included grouping, supper recurrence, period, time inside period, and time duplicate by feast recurrence collaboration as fixed impacts. Period and time were displayed as rehashed measures. The factor subject settled in grouping was remembered for the model as an intermittent impact. The primary perception inside a period was incorporated as a covariate. At the point when the time multiply by dinner recurrence connection was critical (P is equivalent to 0.05), inside time supper recurrence impacts were assessed by utilizing rehashed measures ANOVA. In the event that this collaboration was not huge, the principle impact of dinner recurrence was assessed. Information are introduced as means SEMs.

Characteristics of Subjects

69 people went to the examination data meeting. 35 gave composed educated assent, and 32 finished the screening interaction. 21 subjects (14 ladies, 7 men) at last were haphazardly appointed to the medicines. Fifteen subjects (10 ladies, 5 men) finished the taking care of period of the investigation. Complete information were examined and are introduced for 15 subjects. In the 3 feast/d eating routine arm, 1 subject pulled out in light of food disdains. During the 1 feast/d eating regimen, 5 subjects pulled out in light of booking clashes and medical issues irrelevant to the examination. Just 1 of the 5 subjects pulled out explicitly due to a reluctance to devour the 1 supper/d eating regimen. The mean BMI showed that subjects were inside the ordinary reach. The actual qualities of the 15 subjects at gauge are introduced.

Diet Plans

The sythesis of the 2 weight control plans is appeared. Subject adherence to the controlled eating regimens was decided to be great based on noticed utilization of the suppers in the office and audit of the reactions on the day by day surveys. The intermittent fasting triacylglycerol and glucose focuses demonstrated that consistence with the 1 feast/d eating regimen was worthy. The mean triacylglycerol and glucose fixations were 64.4 and 79.7 mg/dL, individually. Thirty of 1650 evening dinners (1.8%) gave during the whole examination were stuffed for utilization away from the office. The normal day by day energy admission across medicines was 2364 kcal in the 1 dinner/d eating regimen and 2429 kcal in the 3 suppers/d eating routine. No huge contrasts were found in the rates of macronutrients, unsaturated fats, cholesterol, and fiber between the 2 controlled eating regimens.

Blood Pressure

Systolic and diastolic blood pressures were essentially brought down by 6% during the period when subjects were devouring 3 dinners/d than when they were burning-through 1 supper/day. No critical impact of time (estimations taken at week 4 and week 8) or of treatment arrangement on circulatory strain was seen. No critical contrasts in pulse and internal heat level were seen between the 2 eating routine regimens.

Scales of Visual Analogue

There was a huge treatment impact between the 2 weight control plans on evaluations of appetite, want to eat, completion, and forthcoming utilization (i.e., the measure of food subjects figured they could eat). The 1 dinner/d eating routine was altogether higher for hunger (P is equivalent to 0.003), want to eat (P is equivalent to 0.004), and planned utilization (P is equivalent to 0.006) than was the 3 suppers/d eating regimen. Sensations of completion were essentially (P is equivalent to 0.001) lower in the 1 feast/day than in the 3 dinners/day diet. Notwithstanding the huge treatment impact by diet, a huge time impact (day of study) was noticed for hunger, want to eat, totality, and imminent utilization. Over the long run, hunger, want to eat, and imminent utilization were fundamentally higher in the 1 dinner/day than in the 3 suppers/day diet. Completion was fundamentally lower over the long run in the 1 supper/day diet than in the 3 dinners/day diet.

Body Composition and Weight

Subjects' weight and muscle versus fat mass were brought down (1.4 and 2.1 kg, separately) after utilization of the 1 supper/day diet yet not after utilization of the 3 dinners/day diet. No critical contrasts in sans fat mass and complete body water were seen between the eating routine gatherings. Indeed, even with an 11-week waste of time period between the 2 eating routine conventions, no critical contrasts from benchmark were found in body weight, fat mass, sans fat mass, or complete body water in one or the other time of the investigation. No proof was found of a critical contrast in active work after utilization of the 1 supper/day or the 3 dinners/day diet.

Biological Samples

Utilization of 1 dinner/day brought down blood urea nitrogen by 13.4%. The serum liver proteins antacid phosphatase, serum glutamic pyruvic transaminase, and serum glutamic oxaloacetic transaminase were higher 4.6%, 17.5%, and 16.0% higher, individually, when subjects devoured 1 feast/day than when they burned-through 3 dinners/d. Serum egg whites was 4.5% higher and cortisol fixations were 48.9% lower after utilization of 1 dinner/day than after utilization of 3 suppers/day. Aggregate, LDL, and HDL cholesterol were 11.7%, 16.8%, and 8.4% higher, separately, in subjects devouring 1 supper/day than in those burning-through 3 dinners/day. The hematologic factors that contrasted altogether between the eating regimens bunches were those of hemoglobin, hematocrit and red platelets. Serum convergences of creatinine, glucose, complete protein, uric corrosive, and any remaining metabolic factors were not essentially influenced by the weight control plans.

2.4 Discussion

This investigation is among the main controlled randomized clinical preliminaries to assess the impacts of controlled feast recurrence on ordinary weight, moderately aged grown-ups. We tracked down that the utilization of a dinner skipping diet (i.e., 1 supper/day), instead of the customary 3 dinners/day diet, is attainable for a brief length.

Our examination withdrawal rate was 28.6%. Commonplace paces of withdrawal from human taking care of studies at our office are 4–7% (18–20). We can estimate that subject withdrawals expanded on the grounds that the subjects were approached to devour all nourishment for the day in 1 dinner; nonetheless, just 1 subject explicitly expressed this justification pulling out. Most subjects had the option to burn-through all calories in the 1 feast/day diet. Study withdrawals were accounted for to be because of subject booking clashes and medical conditions that were irrelevant to the investigation.

A couple of exploratory investigations have tried the impact of feast recurrence on satiety measures. The aftereffects of the VASs recommend that subjects didn't get acclimated to the 1 dinner/day diet. Over the long run, hunger, want to eat, and forthcoming utilization expanded, while sensations of completion diminished. Essentially, subjects who followed another day-fasting diet for multi week had a critical expansion in craving and want to eat on their fasting days than at gauge, however they didn't get acclimated to the other day-fasting diet, and they were similarly as eager on their first day of fasting as on the most recent day. Albeit abstract craving and satiety evaluations were not made after the evening supper, in remarks during utilization of the 1 feast/day diet, most subjects detailed limit totality after the dinner and experienced issues completing their food in the assigned time. Further exploration is needed to acquire a superior comprehension of emotional satiety on dinner recurrence.

In spite of the fact that inside typical qualities, both systolic and diastolic blood pressures were higher than pattern during utilization of the 1 feast/day diet. Trial information for typical weight people on the impacts of utilization of 1 feast/day instead of 3 dinners/day on pulse have not recently been accounted for. Overweight people showed that utilization of 1 supper/day, with caloric limitation, improved circulatory strain and pulse after work out. In creature models, intermittent fasting without caloric limitation has been appeared to diminish pulse and pulse. The noticed expansion in pulse in our subject populace burning-through 1 feast/day might be because of a circadian cadence in circulatory strain. Diurnal changes may have happened, in light of the fact that pulse estimations were acquired in the late evening in the 1 dinner/d eating routine versus early morning in the 3 suppers/day.

It is fascinating that body weight and muscle versus fat diminished in the 1 supper/day diet, which might be mostly clarified by a slight shortfall of 65 kcal in day by day energy admission. This adjustment of body organization may likewise be impacted by the impact that eating examples could have on metabolic action. Subjects that followed a snacking diet and afterward an eating routine that comprising of 1 enormous dinner built up an expansion net transition of free unsaturated fats from fat stores and an increment in gluconeogenesis. Comparable changes in digestion may have happened in our subjects, which may have added to weight and fat mass misfortune. Gluconeogenesis ordinarily starts 4–6 hours after the last feast and turns out to be completely dynamic as stores of liver glycogen are exhausted. Free unsaturated fats and amino acids that are substrates for gluconeogenesis are utilized for the energy supply.

Adjusted coursing lipid focuses are perceived as hazard factors for CVD. In the current investigation, we found both (expansions altogether and LDL cholesterol) and (an increment in HDL cholesterol and a reduction in triacylglycerols) changes after utilization of the 1 dinner/day diet. These progressions gave off an impression of being autonomous of the controlled eating regimens, since dietary cholesterol and the proportion of unsaturated fats were held steady. Studies that have endeavored to decide the impacts of supper recurrence on biomarkers of wellbeing, like lipid focuses, are conflicting. In one exploratory investigation, sound men were taken care of either 3 dinners/day or 17 little bites/d for multi week; subjects burning-through the 17-nibble diet had decreases altogether and LDL-cholesterol fixations, while the focuses didn't change in the subjects burning-through 3 suppers/day. Two examinations likewise showed that excluding breakfast effect wellbeing results identified with CVD, and another investigation showed that this exclusion may diminish hazard factors for CVD.

Utilization of 1 feast/d expanded egg whites and liver catalysts and diminished blood urea nitrogen in our examination subjects, albeit these qualities stayed inside typical reference ranges. Subjects burning-through the 1 feast/d eating regimen additionally had diminished cortisol focuses. Albeit all blood assortment happened following 12 hours of fasting, the circumstance of blood assortment contrasted between the 2 eating regimen gatherings. Blood was gathered in the early morning, before breakfast (i.e., following a 12 hours quick), from subjects burning-through 3 suppers/day and in the late evening, before the evening feast (i.e., following a 18-hours quick), from those burning-through I dinner/day. Subjects burning-through 1 dinner/day had diminished cortisol fixations, which were in all probability because of diurnal varieties in this chemical. Cortisol is ordinarily raised in the first part of the day and diminishes later in the early evening.

During Ramadan, the heavenly month during which Muslims quick from day break to nightfall, diurnal varieties of nourishment biomarkers have been seen in rehearsing Muslims. Past research has shown that, dissimilar to in non-fasting periods, cortisol focuses are biphasic during Ramadan fasting. These specialists announced an increment in serum cortisol beginning at 1200 hours that arrives at a level somewhere in the range of 1600 and 2000. During Ramadan fasting, diurnal variety in cortisol varies altogether from the ordinary diurnal variety. We found that subjects' hemoglobin, hematocrit, and red platelets were lower after utilization of the 1 supper/day diet, while the mean cell volume was viewed as of ordinary focus. The last outcomes could be the consequence of an expansion in blood volume or an adjustment of the creation of red platelets. Past research on Ramadan fasting has shown a concealment in red platelet creation alongside an expanding pattern for pallor. The last outcomes were likely because of a reduction in the admissions of calories and of iron-containing food varieties during the fasting month of Ramadan. No major, clinically pertinent, diet-related changes were found in the exhaustive metabolic board or CBC, which demonstrated that the 1 dinner/day diet was very much endured in that gathering of solid people.

A few impediments of the plan of the current examination warrant thought. Albeit this was a pilot study, the little example size was especially restricting. Blood, circulatory strain, internal heat level, and body-piece estimations were taken in the early morning from subjects devouring 3 dinners/day and in the late evening from those burning-through l feast/day; results may have varied if the last estimations additionally were gotten in the early morning. BIA may likewise not be the best technique for evaluating body organization due to its inclination to overestimate fat mass in fit subjects. The subject populace of the flow concentrate additionally was genuinely homogenous; future exploration ought to incorporate overweight and stout populaces to permit assurance of the impacts of feast recurrence in those gatherings.

Past examinations archived enhancements in the wellbeing and life span of subjects and subject kept up on an intermittent fasting routine wherein they were denied of nourishment for a 24-hours' time frame each and every day; in these investigations, the test diet brought about by and large decreases in calorie admission of up to 30%. Nonetheless, in certain investigations, the measure of caloric limitation was little (5–10%) and the physiologic changes were generally huge, which recommends that the all-inclusive fasting period itself added to the advantages of the eating regimen. The current discoveries propose that, without a decrease in calorie consumption, a diminished dinner recurrence diet doesn't bear the cost of significant medical advantages in people. Enhancements in glucose guideline and cardiovascular wellbeing in subjects happen during a while of intermittent fasting; the time during which the subjects were kept up on the 1 supper/day diet in the current investigation may in this manner not be adequate to accomplish stable changes in physiology. A drawn out diminished dinner recurrence diet that likewise remembers a 20–30% decrease for calorie admission would all the more intently look like the intermittent fasting routine that is broadly utilized in rat contemplates.

Taking everything into account, changed supper recurrence is possible in sound, typical weight, moderately aged people. Utilization of 1 supper/day brought about weight reduction and a lessening in fat mass with little alteration in calorie utilization. It stays indistinct whether adjusted feast recurrence would prompt changes in weight and body synthesis in large subjects.

Conclusion

Typical weight subjects can conform to a 1 feast/day eating routine. At the point when feast recurrence is diminished without a decrease in by and large calorie admission, unobtrusive changes happen in body creation, some cardiovascular illness hazard factors, and hematologic factors. Diurnal varieties may influence results. Subjects who finished the investigation kept up their body weight inside 2 kg of their underlying load all through the 6-month period. There were no huge impacts of supper recurrence on pulse, internal heat level, or a large portion of the blood factors estimated. Be that as it may, while burning-through 1 feast/day, subjects had a huge expansion in hunger; a critical adjustment of body piece, remembering decreases for fat mass; huge expansions in pulse and altogether, LDL-, and HDL-cholesterol focuses; and a huge abatement in convergences of cortisol.

Lightning Source UK Ltd.
Milton Keynes UK
UKHW020642240521
384271UK00011B/796